Introductory Statistics for Health and Nursing Using SPSS

COMPANION WEBSITE

Visit the companion website at www.uk.sagepub.com/ marston to find datasets and additional questions.

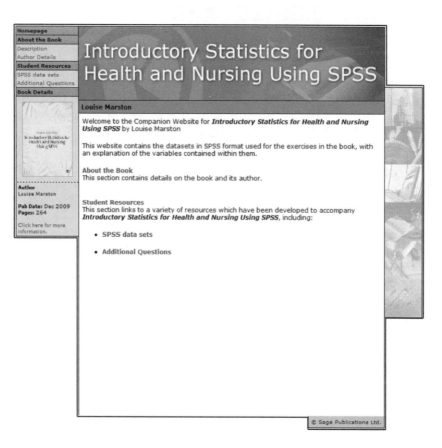

Introductory Statistics for Health and Nursing Using SPSS

Louise Marston

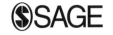

Los Angeles | London | New Delhi
Singapore | Washington DC

First published 2010

SAGE Publications Ltd
1 Oliver's Yard
55 City Road
London EC1Y 1SP

SAGE Publications Inc.
2455 Teller Road
Thousand Oaks, California 91320

SAGE Publications India Pvt Ltd
B 1/I 1 Mohan Cooperative Industrial Area
Mathura Road
New Delhi 110 044

SAGE Publications Asia-Pacific Pte Ltd
33 Pekin Street #02-01
Far East Square
Singapore 048763

Library of Congress Control Number: 2009927204

British Library Cataloguing in Publication data

A catalogue record for this book is available from the British Library

ISBN 978-1-84787-482-5
ISBN 978-1-84787-483-2 (pbk)

Typeset by C&M Digitals (P) Ltd, Chennai, India
Printed by MPG Books Group, Bodmin, Cornwall
Printed on paper from sustainable resources

Mixed Sources
Product group from well-managed forests and other controlled sources
www.fsc.org Cert no. SA-COC-1565
© 1996 Forest Stewardship Council
FSC

For my father, Roger Marston
and
my mother, Joy Marston.

CONTENTS

PREFACE

This book came about through teaching MSc students in nursing and other health related disciplines, where I found there was no book that described the statistics I was teaching and set it with SPSS whilst giving examples related to health. This book assumes no knowledge of SPSS or statistics, and starts by describing features of data before introducing SPSS and then combines the two with data entry and management. As background to the research process, study designs and the concepts of samples and populations are explained and illustrated using published literature. Chapter 4, the final background chapter, is on probability, showing how simple concepts work before linking probability to health statistics. This book continues by describing the statistical techniques and tests commonly taught to students of nursing and other health related disciplines – both undergraduate and postgraduate. It gives examples of how each technique and test is carried out using SPSS. Each example shown uses data from real studies; some of which were collected by the students I taught. Real data are important because they show the patterns and deviations that students may see in their datasets. There are exercises at the end of each chapter so that students can test their understanding of the chapter. Some of the exercises are designed to be used with SPSS by analysing the data; giving practice with SPSS, data analysis and interpretation of the results.

I would like to express my thanks to Kiran Katikaneni, Carol Morant, Mathew Alfred, Maria Stein and Aminollah Ferdowsian for allowing me to use their data in this book. Also thank you to Alison Sherwin for allowing me to use a screenshot of her variable names. I would also like to thank Janet Peacock for allowing me to use data we have both been very close to for a number of years, and also for encouraging me to write the book. Finally, thank you to Julie Gilg and Gita Thakur for reading the book; and for spotting inconsistencies and typos. However, any that remain are my own.

Louise Marston
February 2009

1
GETTING STARTED WITH DATA AND SPSS

INTRODUCTION

When undertaking research studies, it is likely that data will have been collected. Much of this will be in a form suitable to be analysed statistically; that is, responses from a questionnaire or data collection sheet can be coded so that each response is represented by a number. When data have been coded, it can be entered to a data analysis program such as SPSS. SPSS is menu driven, making it easy to use.

This chapter will start by distinguishing between types of data. It will then move onto the situation of a pile of questionnaires that need to be coded before data are entered into SPSS. It will show the conventions for assigning codes to questionnaires before the data entry process. It will then go onto opening SPSS and giving a tour of features that will be explained during the course of this book. This will lead to how to set up a datasheet so that data can be entered into SPSS. The chapter then moves onto saving data and an introduction to SPSS syntax, which is mainly used as a means of recording the commands used for future analysis. Finally, actions associated with closing SPSS, encompassing saving, printing and exporting output are explained.

This chapter uses a questionnaire asking hotel employees about their knowledge of diabetes as well as the data collected from the resulting study.

THE AIMS OF THIS CHAPTER ARE:

- To distinguish between types of data.
- To learn how to code questionnaires/data collection sheets so the resulting data can be entered into SPSS.
- To show how to open SPSS.
- To guide the user round the windows and menus that comprise SPSS, so that data can be opened, entered and ultimately analysed.
- To explain how to save data, output and command syntax.

PRELIMINARY TO THIS CHAPTER

This ⊙ is a radio button. SPSS uses them when it requires one option to be selected.

TYPES OF DATA

Paramount to all data entry and analysis is the knowledge of what type of data a given variable is because different types of data are coded and ultimately analysed in different ways. SPSS gives three options regarding types of data: nominal, ordinal and scale.

Nominal data

These are categorical data that have no order. The categories within each variable are mutually exclusive: respondents can only fall into one category. For example, respondents can only be one ethnicity from a given list. Where a nominal variable has two categories, it is often referred to as dichotomous or binary.

Examples of nominal variables:

> Gender – respondents can be male or female
> Disease/health status – respondents can either have a disease or not
> Marital status – respondents can only have one marital status at a given time: single, married, separated, divorced, widowed

Ordinal data

These are also categorical variables in which the categories are ordered.

Examples of ordinal variables:

> Age group – for example, 30–39, 40–49, 50–59, 60+
> Likert scales – strongly agree, agree, neither agree nor disagree, disagree, strongly disagree

Scale data

In SPSS this covers discrete and continuous data. Discrete data comprise variables that can only take integers (whole numbers).

Examples of discrete data:

> Number of nights spent in hospital
> Number of courses of a given drug prescribed during the study period
> Age at last birthday
> Number of cigarettes smoked in a week

Continuous data can (in theory at least) take any value. However, this is usually restricted by the accuracy of the equipment used for measuring. For example, scales for weighing adult human weights rarely measure more accurately than whole kilograms and occasionally to one decimal place. This is also for practical reasons; there is little need to weigh adult humans to greater precision than the nearest kilogram or 100 grams (1 decimal place).

Examples of continuous data:

> Blood pressure
> Body mass index (BMI)
> Lung function, for example peak expiratory flow rate (PEFR)

CODING QUESTIONNAIRES

Once data collection is complete, then the next task is to decide how to code each question so that it can easily be seen which values should be inputted into SPSS. This is necessary because numerical values are needed representing answers to questions on a questionnaire or other data collection sheet for SPSS to analyse the data. The initial task of deciding on coding is best done using an unused questionnaire so that all possible codes can be written on the questionnaire without confusion. In addition, it is a good idea to write the variable names on this questionnaire. These steps help the coding process so that individual codes do not have to be remembered and also provides a permanent record of the coding of the dataset.

Figures 1.1a, 1.1b and 1.1c show excerpts from a questionnaire aimed at hotel employees to discover their knowledge of diabetes and to find out whether employees consider hotels (as a workplace) to be appropriate places to conduct health promotion specifically aimed at type 2 diabetes. These excerpts have not been annotated with possible variable names, but have been annotated with coding. Variable names should not be long (ideally eight characters), but should be as descriptive as possible (when setting up an SPSS datasheet it is possible to give each variable a longer label, this will be explained later in this chapter). Variable names must be unique within a dataset.

Questions 2 and 3 (Figure 1.1a) produced nominal data; there is no ordering. Question 2 lists three options and participants were asked to select one, therefore a different code is needed for all options. As the data are nominal the numbers given

2. To the best of your knowledge can diabetes type 2 be delayed?

○ Yes   1
○ No   2
○ Don't know   3

3. Which of the following do you recognise as symptoms of diabetes type 2? (tick all that apply)

☐ Tiredness   1   ☐ Excessive thirst   1
☐ Tension and depression   1   ☐ Loss of weight   1
☐ Frequent urination   1   ☐ Giddiness   1
☐ Slow healing of wounds   1   ☐ Excessive hunger   1

FIGURE 1.1A EXCERPT FROM A QUESTIONNAIRE – QUESTIONS GIVING NOMINAL DATA

10. Please state your weight in either kgs, lbs or stones and your height in cm or inches.

                Weight   Height

Weight in kgs, lbs, stns; Height in cm or inches   [▼]   [▼]

FIGURE 1.1B EXCERPT FROM A QUESTIONNAIRE – QUESTIONS GIVING CONTINUOUS DATA

as the codes do not necessarily have to be 1, 2 and 3, they could have equally been 0, 1, and 2 or any other three unique numbers. The convention is to code nominal data using consecutive numbers, starting with 0 or 1.

Question 3 allows the participant to select as many options as they want. Therefore, each potential response needs to be coded and entered as a separate variable. Therefore, although it is presented on the questionnaire as one question, when the data are entered into SPSS for analysis, there will be eight variables. With Question 3, if the participant has not selected a given option, it is assumed that they do not recognise that option as a symptom of type 2 diabetes so these are eight yes and no questions. The simplest way to code these is to code as 1 where the option has been selected and 0 otherwise, giving coding of $0 = $ no and $1 = $ yes.

Question 10 (Figure 1.1b) gives scale data. It requires the participant to put their actual height and weight in the two boxes provided (data for this study were collected through an online questionnaire so there were dropdown menus giving possible options). If the questionnaire was completed using a pen and paper, it would be advantageous to put the possible units beside the measure and instruct the participant to select the units they are giving their measurements in. The number of variables equal to the number of types of units used would be entered into SPSS. For example, with height, there may be two variables: height in metres and height in inches. Exact heights and weights would be entered into SPSS. Conversion into one set of units for each variable would take place using SPSS to ensure there are no human errors resulting from the calculations being done by hand.

12. Questions 12–16 ask about your opinion of health promotion programmes in the workplace. Please select the option that best represents your view.

	Believe strongly	Believe slightly	Not sure	Believe a little	Not at all
My company should help create greater awareness about diabetes prevention at work.	○	○	○	○	○
My workplace is a suitable environment for promoting diabetes prevention awareness programmes.	○	○	○	○	○
	1	2	3	4	5

FIGURE 1.1C   EXCERPT FROM A QUESTIONNAIRE – QUESTIONS GIVING ORDINAL DATA

The questions in Figure 1.1c use likert scales in which participants are asked to select the response closest to their opinion. The possible responses are ordered through the spectrum of opinions. The responses range from 'believe strongly' to 'not at all' with a neutral category in the middle. As these options are ordered, the codes that will be entered into SPSS should also be ordered. Therefore, in this example, the responses are coded from 1 to 5.

Further information

For more information on coding see Chapter 2 of Peacock and Kerry (2007).

OPENING SPSS

Now there are some data to put into SPSS, the program can be opened. To do this, click on Start → Programs → SPSS for Windows → SPSS for Windows. When this has been done, the initial screen will appear. An example of this can be seen in Figure 1.2. A window appears on top of the SPSS Data Editor. If the data file required has been used recently, it will appear in the box containing recently used data files. Otherwise click Cancel → File → Open → Data… → find the data file required from where it was last saved. The file name will end .sav.

The Status Bar is the section at the bottom of the screen that usually says SPSS Processor is ready (Figure 1.2). This can be turned off by clicking on View → Status Bar.

When the dataset is open, the SPSS Data Editor will look similar to Figure 1.3. This is Data View. All variables have been coded to numbers. Each row represents a different participant.

Click on the Variable View tab at the bottom left of the screen (indicated in Figure 1.3), to get a screen like Figure 1.4. This is the screen where category codes and missing data codes can be viewed or declared to SPSS. In Figure 1.4 it can be seen that there is one row for each variable in the dataset. The meaning of each of the columns in Variable View and what should be placed in them will be shown later in this chapter in the section on entering data.

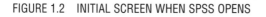

The box where recently used data files will be shown

The box where other recently used files (for example, syntax or output) will be shown

Status bar

FIGURE 1.2   INITIAL SCREEN WHEN SPSS OPENS

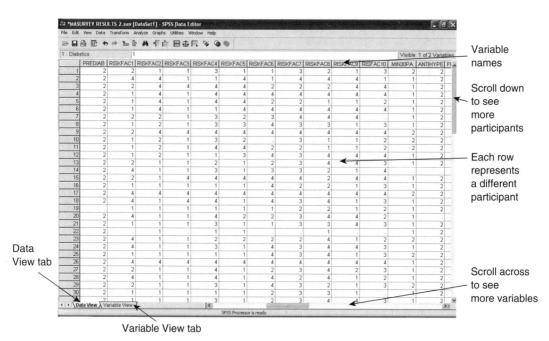

Variable names

Scroll down to see more participants

Each row represents a different participant

Data View tab

Variable View tab

Scroll across to see more variables

FIGURE 1.3   DATA VIEW

A TOUR OF THE SPSS DATA VIEW MENUS AND TOOLBAR

This section will explain options under the SPSS menus which are likely to be used by health scientists and nurses. If an explanation on using any other options within these menus is needed, the built in Help gives information on all functions and commands within SPSS.

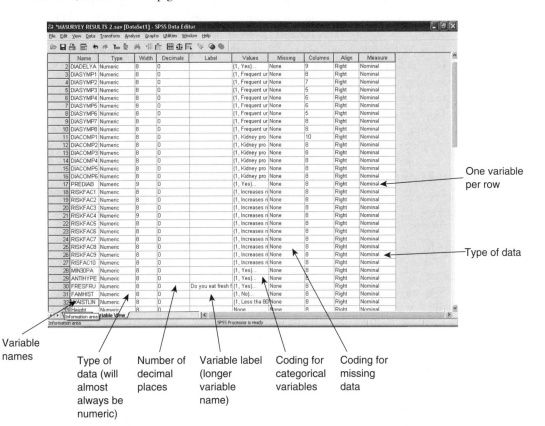

FIGURE 1.4   VARIABLE VIEW

FIGURE 1.5   DATA VIEW SHOWING THE CONTENTS OF THE FILE MENU

File

- Options available under the File menu are shown in Figure 1.5. Many of the options under this menu are similar to those found in other Windows based programs: New, Open, Save, Save As…, Print Preview, Print and Exit.
- Open Database invokes an interface that allows data from a database such as Microsoft Access to be opened directly into SPSS. Likewise, Read Text Data… allows data stored in text formats to be opened.
- Mark File Read Only is used for data protection purposes, so that datasets cannot be modified or deleted. If it is necessary to change the dataset whilst this is in operation, it has to be resaved using a different name. Alternately it is possible to reverse the permissions using Mark file Read Write from the File Menu.
- Display Data File Information shows information about the dataset in the SPSS Viewer (the SPSS Viewer is explained later in this chapter). This includes: the Variable name, Position in the dataset, Label, Measurement Level, Column Width, Alignment, Print Format, Write Format, Missing Values, Value and Label. Most of this information is available in Variable View (Figure 1.4).
- Recently Used Data and Recently Used Files allow datasets or files (output or syntax) that have been opened recently to be opened easily without having to browse directories to find the dataset or file required.

Edit

- This menu (Figure 1.6) largely includes the editing options that are available in other Windows based programs. An additional option is Paste Variables…. Paste Variables… allows exact copies of variables to be created in Variable View. This is useful when a dataset has a number of variables that have similar attributes; variables can be copied and the necessary minor changes made. For example if weight was collected at three time points, the variable attributes can be copied and the variable names and labels changed to make them unique and reflect the three time points.
- Insert Variable and Insert Case allow the user to insert another variable or set of data from a participant into the dataset respectively. These need not necessarily be at the end of the dataset.
- Options… allow the user to change a number of attributes of SPSS, customising to their own preferences.

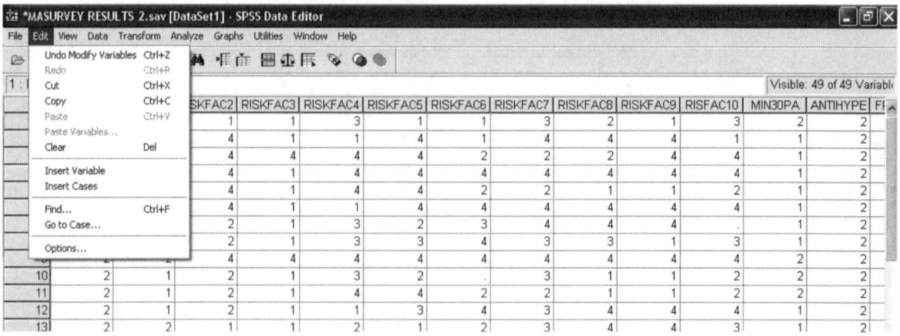

FIGURE 1.6   DATA VIEW SHOWING THE CONTENTS OF THE EDIT MENU

View

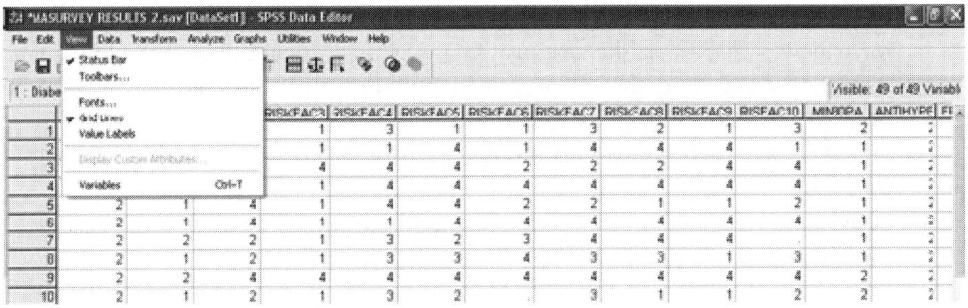

FIGURE 1.7   DATA VIEW SHOWING THE CONTENTS OF THE VIEW MENU

- The icons on the toolbar can be altered using Toolbars....
- The font type and size used in the Data Editor can be changed using Fonts....
- Grid Lines allows the gridlines on Data View to be seen (the default is that they are visible). These can be turned off.
- It is possible to see how the categorical variables have been labelled whilst in Data View by turning Value Labels on.
- When in Data View, clicking on Variables changes the view to Variable View. In Variable View, this menu item is replaced by Data.

Data

- Using the data menu (Figure 1.8), data within a given variable or variables can be sorted using Sort Cases....
- Transpose... creates a new dataset with the rows from the original dataset appearing in the columns and vice versa.

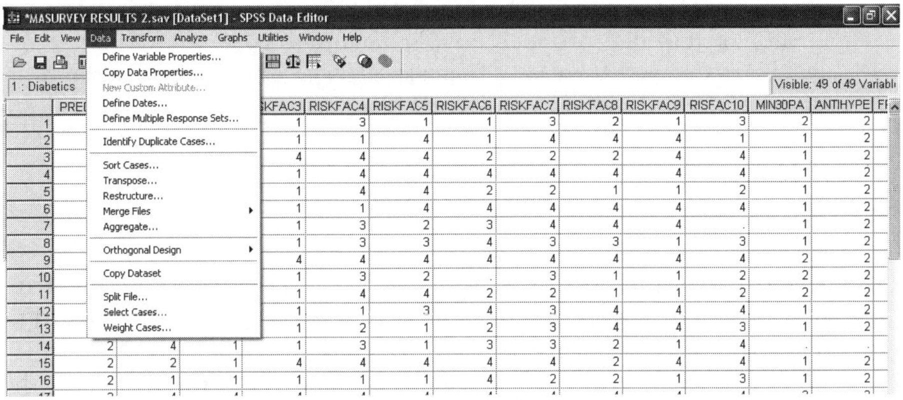

FIGURE 1.8   DATA VIEW SHOWING THE CONTENTS OF THE DATA MENU

- Additional data from another file can be added to the dataset currently open using Merge Files. The data can either be additional participants; in which case at least one of the variable names should be identical (those that are not identical will form new variables in the original dataset). Alternatively, new variables can be added, in which case, the participant identifying variable should be the same in both datasets. This will be explained further in Chapter 2.
- Split File… separates data into groups based on at least one variable for analysis purposes.
- Select Cases… is used if only specific cases (usually defined by specific characteristics) are required. Further explanation on this is in Chapter 2.

Transform

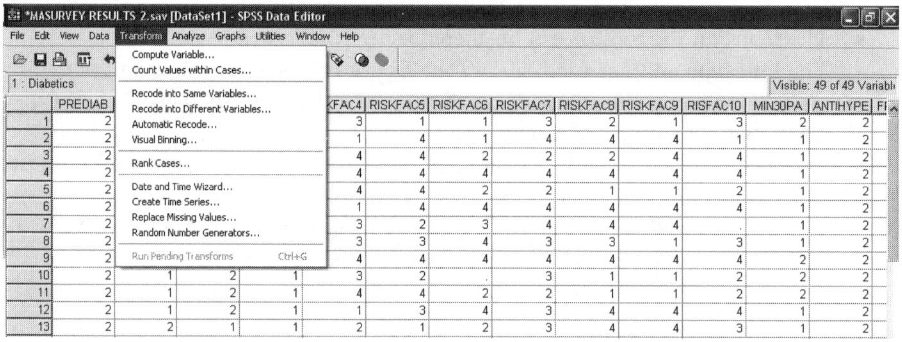

FIGURE 1.9   DATA VIEW SHOWING THE CONTENTS OF THE TRANSFORM MENU

- Compute Variable… is used to generate new variables. These usually utilise SPSS built-in functions such as LN and/or existing variables in the dataset. Details on how to do this will be given in Chapter 2.
- Recode into Same Variables and Recode into Different Variables are used when the coding of variables is altered for analysis, to create coding to transform a continuous variable to a categorical one or to combine responses from more than one variable to create one variable. It may also be used to populate a variable generated using Compute Variable…. Examples of some of these uses are shown in Chapter 2.

Analyze

- All statistical analyses are initiated from the Analyze menu shown in Figure 1.10.
- Reports give elementary case summaries of the dataset. It is more beneficial to summarise the dataset using Descriptive Statistics.
- Descriptive Statistics is used to calculate summary statistics. These will be explained more fully in Chapters 5 and 6.

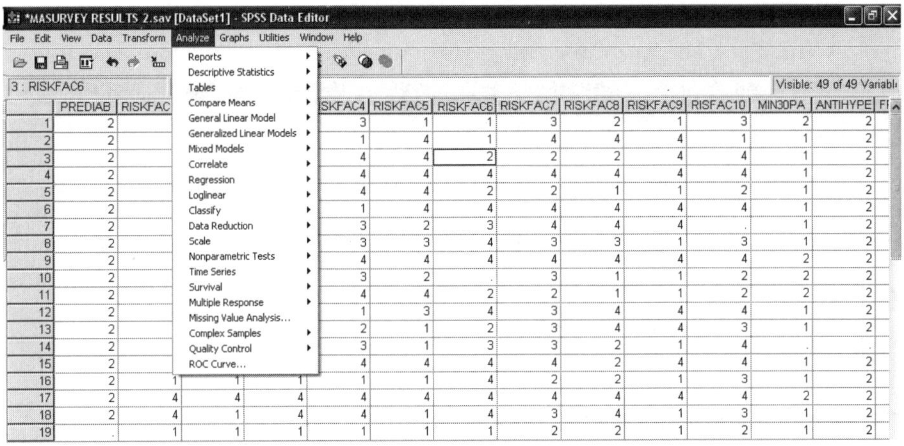

FIGURE 1.10   DATA VIEW SHOWING THE CONTENTS OF THE ANALYZE MENU

- Tables creates tables of summary statistics. Tables of summary statistics can also be created by the levels of categorical variables.
- Compare Means is used to carry out statistical tests that involve the comparison of means, for example, t-tests and one-way ANOVA. These will be discussed in Chapter 9.
- Correlate is used to carry out correlations. These will be explained in Chapter 11.
- Most regression analyses are invoked from the Regression item on the menu. Linear regression and logistic regression will be explained in Chapters 11 and 12.
- All non-parametric tests (for example, Mann–Whitney U test, Wilcoxon Matched Pairs test, Kruskal–Wallis H test) are initiated through the Nonparametric Tests menu item on this menu. An explanation of these will be given in Chapter 10.

Graphs

- The menu shown in Figure 1.11 is the starting point for the production of all stand alone graphics (some graphics can be produced from within specific Analyze menu commands). The easiest way to invoke graphics is to use the Chart Builder.... The use of this will be explained in relation to specific graph types throughout the course of the book.

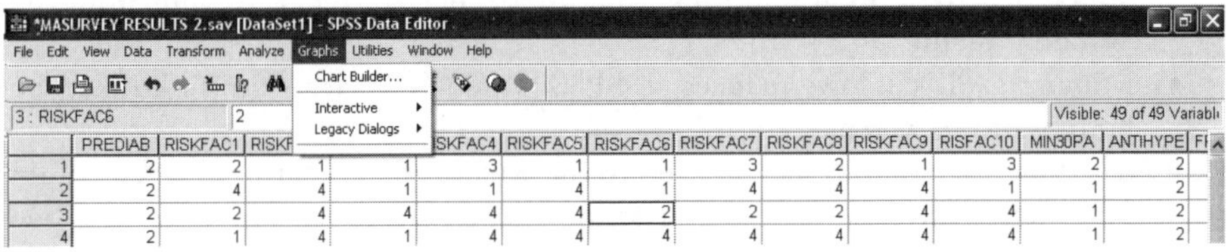

FIGURE 1.11   DATA VIEW SHOWING THE CONTENTS OF THE GRAPHS MENU

Utilities

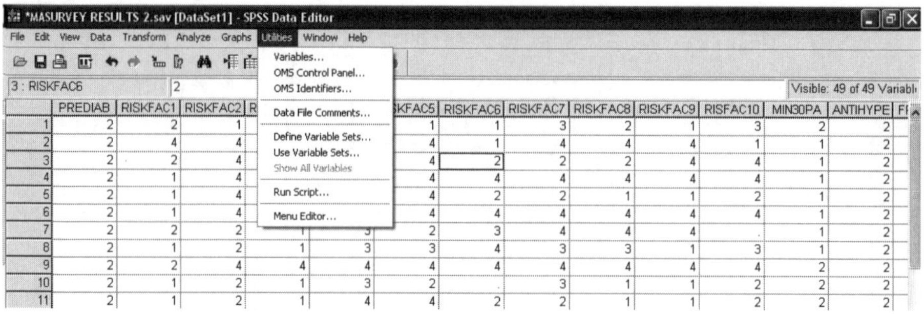

FIGURE 1.12 DATA VIEW SHOWING THE CONTENTS OF THE UTILITIES MENU

- Under the Utilities menu (Figure 1.12), Variables… gives properties, similar to those displayed in Variable View for individual variables. It does not give information for a number of variables simultaneously, so is of limited use.
- Data File Comments… enables the user to add comments about the dataset, which are saved with the dataset. These comments can be shown in the output.

Window

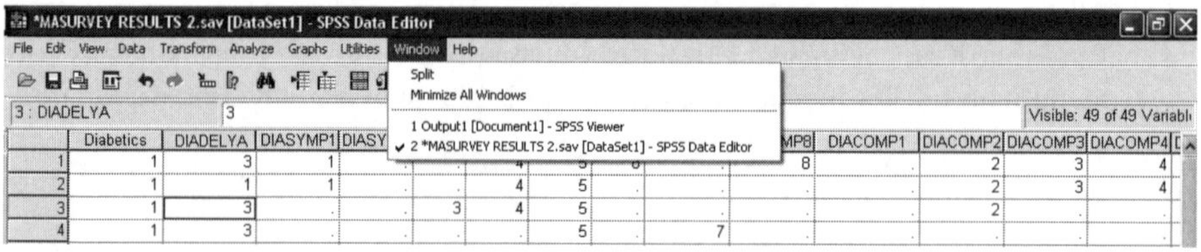

FIGURE 1.13 DATA VIEW SHOWING THE CONTENTS OF THE WINDOW MENU

- Using the Window menu (Figure 1.13), the screen can be divided so that different parts of the dataset can be viewed at the same time using the Split command. The default splits can be moved into positions to suit the user. When the divisions are no longer required, click on Remove Split from the Window menu.
- Minimise All Windows reduces all SPSS windows open to the Taskbar at the bottom of the screen.
- The third item on this menu relates to the window that is currently open within SPSS. When there are a number of windows open it is possible to move from one to another using the list under this menu.

Help

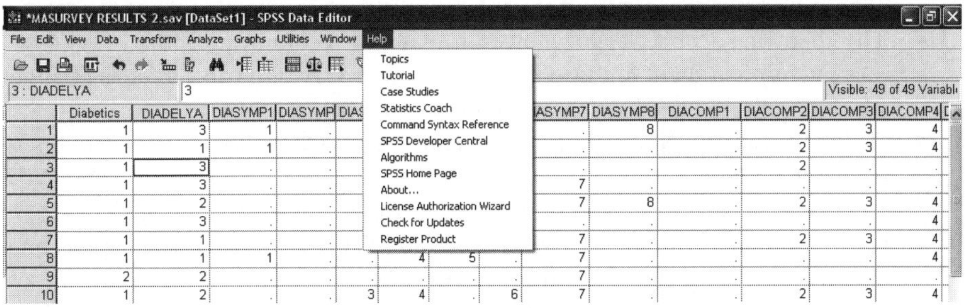

FIGURE 1.14   DATA VIEW SHOWING THE CONTENTS OF THE HELP MENU

- The most useful item on the Help menu (Figure 1.14) is Topics. This performs in a similar way to other Windows based programs.
- Tutorial gives a series of step-by-step guides to a variety of aspects of SPSS including issues related to getting started with SPSS and simple data analysis procedures. Where appropriate the Tutorial is given as a response to the search within Topics.
- Statistics Coach gives basic instructions on what test should be carried out based on the type of data. This function is not a substitute for a good textbook or seeing a statistician.
- Selecting Command Syntax Reference invokes a .pdf document explaining the SPSS syntax.
- Selecting SPSS Home Page invokes an internet browser and then opens the SPSS home page www.spss.com as long as the computer is online.
- About… gives the copyright statement, version number and who the copy of SPSS is licensed to.
- License Authorization Wizard enables the user to give SPSS Inc their authorisation code which locks the copy of SPSS to the hardware.
- Check for Updates connects to www.spss.com to find out whether there are update patches available and if so allows them to be downloaded and installed.
- Register Product enables SPSS to be registered.

Data Editor toolbar

- The data editor toolbar is located underneath the File, Edit, View menus in both Data View and Variable View. This is shown in Figure 1.15.

FIGURE 1.15   DATA EDITOR TOOLBAR

- Starting from the left of Figure 1.15, the first icon is Open File (data).
- The second icon is Save File (greyed out in Figure 1.15). If the data have not previously been saved, Save As is automatically invoked.
- The following icon is Print. However, it is not recommended that the dataset (Data View) is printed because datasets are often very large and inferences about the data will not be able to be made by looking at pages of numbers.
- Dialog Recall displays recently used commands, which can be clicked on to invoke them again.
- Undo and Redo (the left and right pointing arrows, greyed out in Figure 1.15) are used in the same way as with other Microsoft Windows programs. They become usable when an operation has been carried out.
- The icon which resembles a ruler with a red arrow on it is Go To Case. This enables the user to move to a particular case in the dataset. However, this is determined by the grey numbers down the left hand side of Data View rather than any identifying number which may be part of the dataset. Therefore this function has limited use since if the data are sorted, the cases will change in relation to the grey numbers on Data View.
- The following icon is Variables. It enables the user to see much of the information on Variable View variable by variable. This is the same information that can be seen using the Variables command from the Utilities menu.
- The binoculars icon is used for finding particular numbers and/or words within Data View.
- The two icons to the right of Find are Insert Cases and Insert Variable. To use these, highlight a case/variable as required. When the appropriate button is pressed a new case/variable is inserted above/to the left respectively of those already there.
- ▦ is used to split the file, as under the Window menu.
- The scales icon is used to weight cases for statistical analysis. However, for most analyses it will not be necessary to use this function. Weights can also be invoked from the Data menu.
- The first of the final three icons invokes the Value Labels (the same command as that on the View menu), followed by Use Variable Sets and Show All Variables. The final two commands can also be invoked from the Utilities menu.

Opening data saved in formats other than .sav

- Data entered using another program such as Microsoft Excel can be opened in SPSS.
- Click on File → Open → Data... → click on the drop down arrow next to Files of type: to see the types of files that it is possible to open in SPSS (as in Figure 1.16). Choose the format of the file that is required and then locate that file. SPSS will ask for confirmation that the first row contains the variable names and of the length and breadth of the dataset. Then click OK.
- When opening data from some formats (for example, Microsoft Excel), there will be no variable Labels or Values produced. These details can be entered using Variable View.

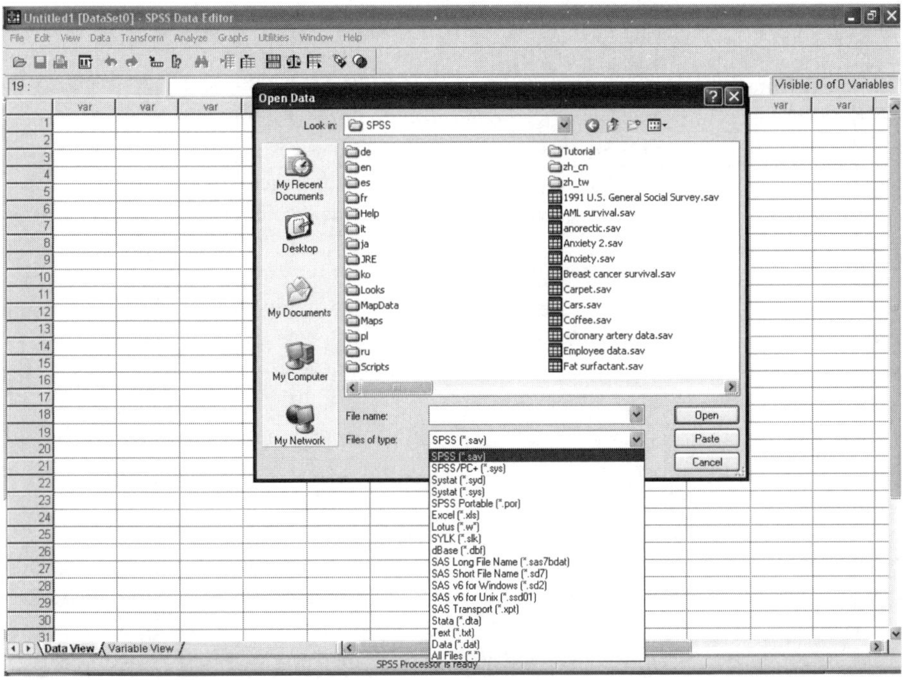

FIGURE 1.16   SCREENSHOT SHOWING THE DATA FORMATS THAT SPSS WILL OPEN

ENTERING DATA

When questionnaires or data extraction sheets have been coded, they are ready to be entered into SPSS.

When SPSS opens, click on the Variable View tab where you will see a screen like Figure 1.17. This screen should be set up to define the variables before data can be entered into Data View.

Name is the variable name, which will appear at the top of columns in Data View. This should be 8 to 10 characters long, and start with an alphanumeric character (letter).

The default for Type is Numeric. This will be appropriate for most data entered into SPSS. Occasionally String (text) or Date (to allow dates to be entered into SPSS) may be needed.

There should be no need to change the Width from the default unless entering text, then this may need to be wider.

Some variables will not need decimal places (for example, the ID number or categorical variables which have been coded). In these circumstances the number of decimal places can be decreased to 0 by either using the arrow in the Decimals cell or typing in the desired number of decimal places, making the data as shown in Data View easier to read. This is shown in Figure 1.18.

Use Label to put in a longer variable name. For example the question as it appears on the questionnaire may be put here. If this is used it will appear in Variables: boxes

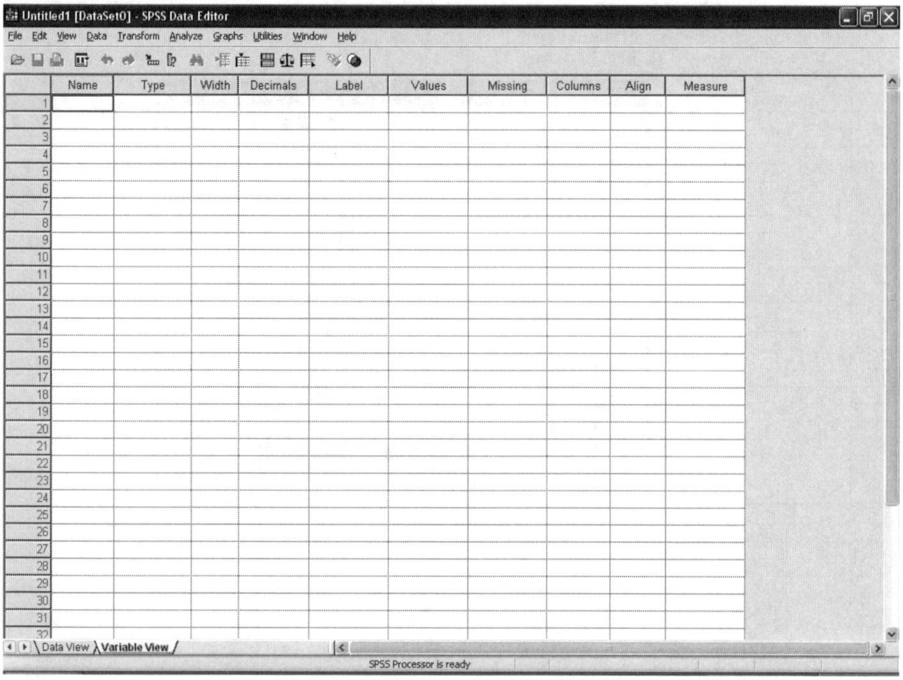

FIGURE 1.17   SCREENSHOT OF VARIABLE VIEW

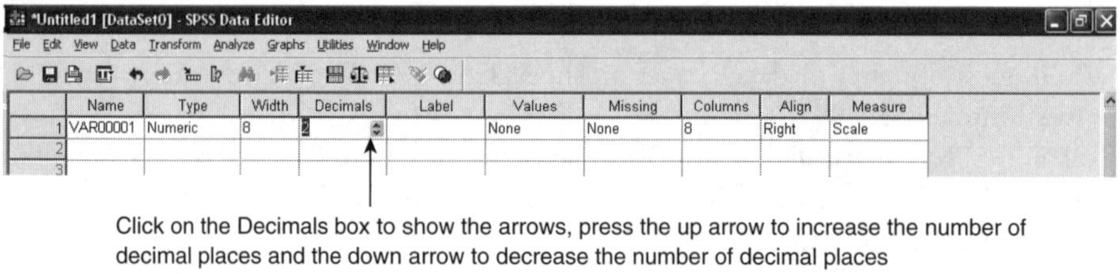

Click on the Decimals box to show the arrows, press the up arrow to increase the number of decimal places and the down arrow to decrease the number of decimal places

FIGURE 1.18   SETTING UP VARIABLE VIEW'S DECIMALS BEFORE ENTERING DATA

alongside the variable name when choosing variables to analyse. It will appear instead of the variable name in some output.

For questions that give nominal or ordinal data, you can tell SPSS how the responses are coded, so that when analyses are carried out, tables and graphics show the textual coding. Click on the Values cell and ... appears in the right of the cell, click on this to get a dialog box like Figure 1.19. In the Value: box put a code for a category of the variable in question, then in the Label: box beneath it, put the category label. When both pieces of information have been added, click Add. Repeat this until all categories within the variable in question have been declared, at which time click OK to return to Variable View (Figure 1.17).

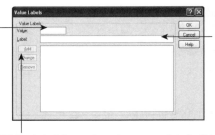

Into the Value: box put the number you are going to use to represent that answer. For example, if yes is going to correspond to 1, put 1 in this box

In the Value Label: box, put what the number in the Value: box represents. For example, to correspond with the 1 in the Value: box, Yes would be typed in this box

When the Value: and Value Label: boxes have been completed, click Add to move them to the large white box. Repeat until all codes have been input. Then click OK

FIGURE 1.19   VALUE LABELS DIALOG BOX

Change the radio button to Discrete missing values, then input up to 3 values which will represent missing data. Then click OK

FIGURE 1.20   MISSING VALUES DIALOG BOX

If the dataset is going to have a specified code for missing data, then the Missing cell should be clicked on. This will give ..., click on this. You will get the dialog box shown in Figure 1.20. The advantage of doing this is that it will be obvious that data for that variable have not been omitted to be entered, and that when entering large amounts of data that are present do not get entered into the wrong cell by not moving to the correct cell. Codes for missing data should not be legal values for the variable in question. For example, if the variable was age of respondent, the value indicating missing should be one that is out of range. There are a number of conventions regarding how missing data are coded. Sometimes columns with missing data are filled with 9, 99, 999 or 9999 depending on possible legal values for the variable. In the age example, the codes for missing values could not be 9 or 99 (depending on the study population), so the most sensible coding for this variable would be 999. Some studies such as the Health Survey for England use negative values to indicate data are missing. The easiest way to declare missing values in the Missing Values dialog box (Figure 1.20) is to click the Discrete missing values radio button, then insert up to three values that indicate missing data. When missing value codes have been declared, click OK to return to Variable View (Figure 1.17).

On Variable View, there should be no need to change the Columns or Align boxes. The Measure column should be changed to match the type of data to be inputted. The default is Scale. This should be used for continuous or discrete data, such as

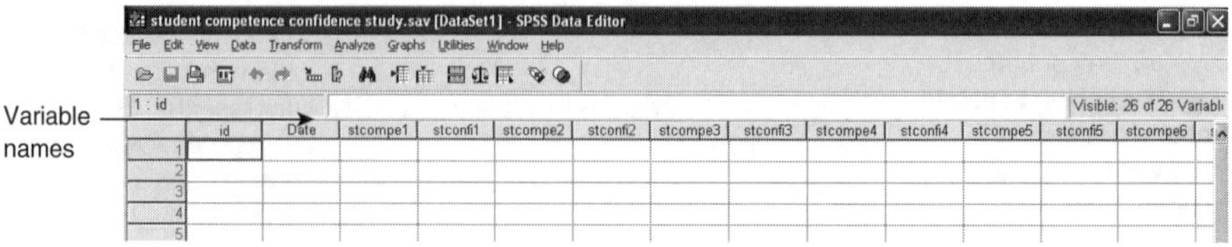

FIGURE 1.21   DATA VIEW WHEN VARIABLE VIEW HAS BEEN SET UP

height or weight. Other options are nominal or ordinal. Variables assigned to these data types should match the descriptions and examples given earlier in this chapter.

The process of setting up the attributes for the variables should be repeated for all variables that will be in the dataset. Once all variables have been defined click on Data View to get a screen like Figure 1.21.

To start entering data, click on the first cell (usually the top left), and begin keying in the data. To move to another cell use the arrow keys on the keyboard (the mouse can also be used, but using the keyboard is quicker). It is easiest to enter all data for each participant before moving on to the next participant.

SAVING DATA

Data will need to be saved. As with other computer programs it is best to do this at regular intervals. In Data View or Variable View click on → File → Save As… and then proceed as for other computer programs.

SPSS VIEWER

All tables, graphics, warnings and information are displayed in the SPSS Viewer (Figure 1.22). The SPSS Viewer opens when SPSS is opened. However, a new SPSS Viewer can be manually opened by clicking on File → New → Output. All subsequent output will be appended to the SPSS Viewer that is open.

Output created in a previous SPSS session can be opened without the relevant dataset being open by clicking on File → Open → Output… → then locating the file required (which will end .spo). If saved output is open and more analysis is carried out, the additional analysis will appear in that SPSS Viewer.

Unwanted output (for example, logs, warnings or results from analyses that are no longer required) can be removed from the SPSS Viewer before it is saved or printed by clicking on the output that is not wanted then pressing delete. Alternately, the item that is no longer required can be located in the Outline Pane and selected. Once selected a box will appear round the item in the main part of the SPSS Viewer; then press delete. Using the Outline Pane is the quickest way of deleting a large number of items from the SPSS Viewer.

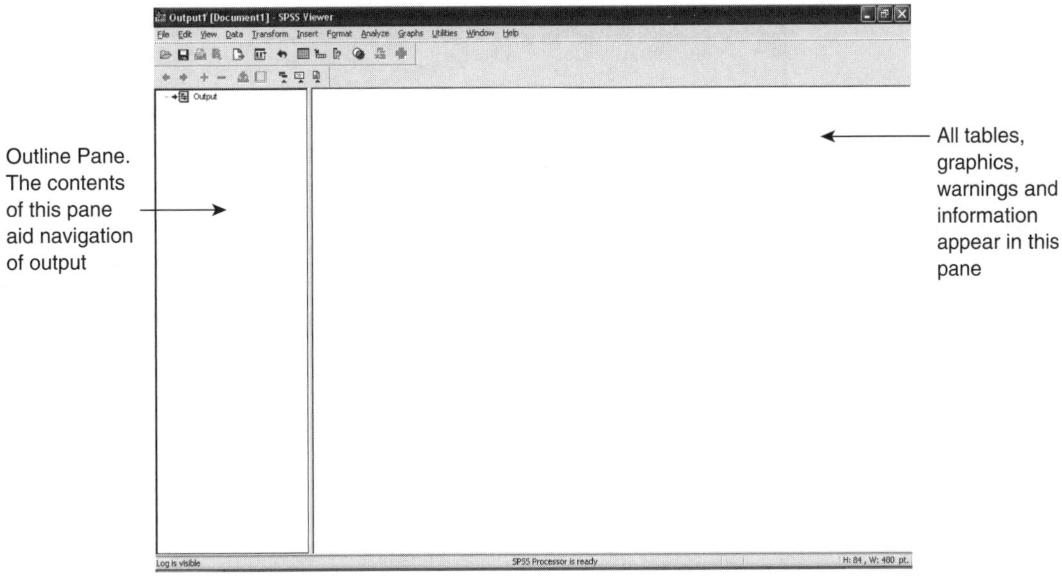

Outline Pane. The contents of this pane aid navigation of output

All tables, graphics, warnings and information appear in this pane

FIGURE 1.22   SPSS VIEWER

PRINTING

It is not recommended that the contents of Data View are printed. The contents of the SPSS Viewer can be printed by clicking on File → Print… when the SPSS Viewer is active. It is possible to print part of the output by highlighting the relevant parts of the Outline Pane.

SAVING OUTPUT

SPSS output can be saved so that the output file can be used later. To do this make sure the SPSS Viewer is open (Figure 1.22). Click on File → Save As… → make sure you save it to where you can retrieve it later. Name your file. Make sure the file type shows as Viewer Files (*.spo), then click OK.

If you want to save the output to read elsewhere, but do not have SPSS, the output can be exported to Microsoft Word or .pdf format. With the SPSS Viewer open, click File → Export this will give a dialog box Figure 1.23. Then select the location and file name of the new document, and the format to export to, before clicking OK.

COPYING OUTPUT TO MICROSOFT WORD

Individual sections of output can be copied and pasted to Microsoft Word. To do this right click with the mouse on the section of output required. This will put a box round it and bring up options such as Cut, Copy and Copy Object. Select Copy

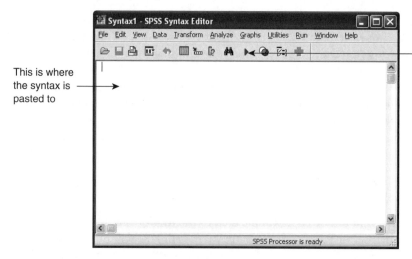

Click on the arrow then choose Output Document, this will include charts too

Put your file name and where you want the document saved to here. Use Browse if you are unsure what the location is called

Click on the arrow and choose Word/RTF (*doc) or Portable Document Format (*.pdf)

Click on OK when all changes are complete

FIGURE 1.23   EXPORT OUTPUT DIALOG BOX

Object. Then open Microsoft Word. At the point where the output is required click the paste icon 📋 (or use Ctrl V) and your selected output will appear.

SYNTAX

SPSS commands can be executed through the drop down menus and pressing OK when the relevant options have been selected. However, it is often necessary to save the commands so that the actions are recorded or the same analysis can be replicated. To use the drop down menus to create syntax, when variables and options have been declared click Paste instead of OK. This will copy the underlying syntax of the command to the SPSS Syntax Editor (Figure 1.24). Syntax can be run by clicking on the arrow indicated in Figure 1.24 or by using the Run drop down menu. Sections of

This is where the syntax is pasted to

This button is used to run the syntax. Sections of syntax can be run by selecting these sections with the mouse

FIGURE 1.24   SYNTAX EDITOR

the syntax can be run by highlighting the required section then clicking the Run arrow or using the Run drop down menu.

Syntax can be saved in the same way as other files (whilst it is explicitly open). This will produce a file with the extension .sps.

When starting a new SPSS session, previous syntax can be reopened by clicking File → Open → Syntax…, then locating the relevant file.

SUMMARY

- Data, output and syntax previously created can be opened through File → Open then choosing the type of file required and then locating the file. Data stored in other formats can be opened in SPSS in a similar way.
- Datasets can be inputted by defining variables using Variable View then inputting data whilst in Data View.
- Individual windows from SPSS can be saved using File → Save As.... To do this, the window required must be active at the time of saving.
- Output can be viewed in Microsoft Word, either by exporting it via File → Export… or by copying and pasting individual tables or graphics to Microsoft Word.
- Commands can be saved by pasting them into the Syntax Editor.

EXERCISES

Below are some survey questions. What type of data would they produce?

1 Do you think the flu vaccine offered this winter protects you from avian flu?

| Yes | ☐ | Don't know | ☐ |
| No | ☐ | Unsure | ☐ |

2 How many times a week do you exercise for more than ½ hour?

Once	☐	Twice	☐
Three times	☐	Four times or more	☐
Never	☐		

3 How old were you when you started smoking? (please fill in your answer).
   _____

Open obesity.sav:

4 How many participants are included in the dataset?
5 How is the variable 'agegroup' coded?

2
DATA MANAGEMENT

INTRODUCTION

Once the data are entered into SPSS, it is inevitable that some degree of data management or manipulation will be necessary before analysing data. It is much better do this using SPSS than 'by hand'. It is inevitable that mistakes, such as errors in entering the data or transposing between columns will occur if data management is done 'by hand'. Moreover, if the dataset is large, carrying out such manipulations will be time consuming. Additionally, if syntax is being utilised, a record of the data management is made so that the process can be replicated in the future and others using the dataset know the logic behind the changes made. Data management functions may include recoding variables that are already present in the dataset, deriving new variables from variables already in the dataset, selecting specific cases for analysis or merging datasets. This chapter includes a number of data management functions that are useful in a variety of circumstances.

This chapter uses data from the student breast cancer awareness study. Data were collected in a cross sectional survey from female staff and students aged less than 50 years at a UK university. This chapter also utilises the student obesity dataset, which asked about risk factors for and opinions on obesity.

THE AIMS OF THIS CHAPTER ARE:

- To demonstrate a number of data management functions within SPSS to enable more succinct data analysis.

PRELIMINARIES TO THIS CHAPTER

Dialog boxes are invoked when the majority of menu items are selected. They allow specific choices related to the procedure to be made.

This arrow ⊡ is used by SPSS to transfer variables or functions around dialog boxes.

RECODING VARIABLES

Sometimes it may be necessary to recode variables. For example, it may be necessary to collapse categories within a variable. For example, ethnicity may have been collected in more categories that it is practical to use for analysis. Alternately, numerical codes may need changing to facilitate statistical modelling. For example, when doing logistic regression (described further in Chapter 12), the dependent (outcome) variable should be coded 0 versus 1, but may not have been coded so when data were originally entered. Recoding can also be used to categorise a variable which was collected as a continuous variable, but will be analysed as a categorical variable. For example, BMI score may be categorised to underweight, normal range, overweight and obese using standard cut-offs.

When recoding, it is advisable to recode into a new variable so that the original variable can still be used if necessary.

For example, using the student breast cancer awareness survey, ethnicity was collected in a large number of categories. For analysis purposes, it is beneficial to recode these to three categories: 'white', 'black' and 'other' because some of the categories had very small frequencies within them (for example, there was only one Bangladeshi woman), therefore it would be difficult to make inferences about those groups. The original variable was coded as shown in Figure 2.1.

To recode data into a different variable click on Transform → Recode into Different Variables … to get the Recode into Different Variables dialog box shown in Figure 2.2.

The variable to be recoded should be transferred to the Input Variable → Output Variable: box and a new variable name declared in the Output Variable Name: box. It is also possible (although not compulsory, this can also be done in Variable View

Ethnicity

		Frequency	Percent	Valid Percent	Cumulative Percent
Valid	White British	61	37.7	38.9	38.9
	White Irish	1	.6	.6	39.5
	White other	3	1.9	1.9	41.4
	Black British	22	13.6	14.0	55.4
	Black Caribbean	11	6.8	7.0	62.4
	Black African	13	8.0	8.3	70.7
	Mixed (B&W)	6	3.7	3.8	74.5
	Mixed other	3	1.9	1.9	76.4
	Indian	14	8.6	8.9	85.4
	Pakistani	4	2.5	2.5	87.9
	Bangladeshi	1	.6	.6	88.5
	Chinese	6	3.7	3.8	92.4
	Other	12	7.4	7.6	100.0
	Total	157	96.9	100.0	
Missing	System	5	3.1		
Total		162	100.0		

FIGURE 2.1   FREQUENCIES OF ETHNICITIES OF WOMEN WHO PARTICIPATED IN A BREAST AWARENESS SURVEY

Note: further explanation of frequencies is given in Chapters 5 and 6.

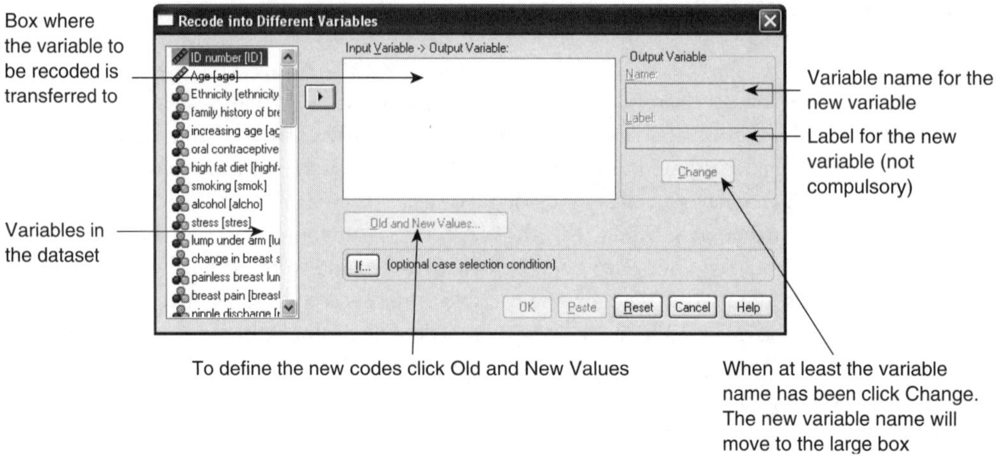

Box where
the variable to
be recoded is
transferred to

Variables in
the dataset

Variable name for the
new variable

Label for the new
variable (not
compulsory)

To define the new codes click Old and New Values

When at least the variable
name has been click Change.
The new variable name will
move to the large box

FIGURE 2.2   RECODE INTO DIFFERENT VARIABLES DIALOG BOX

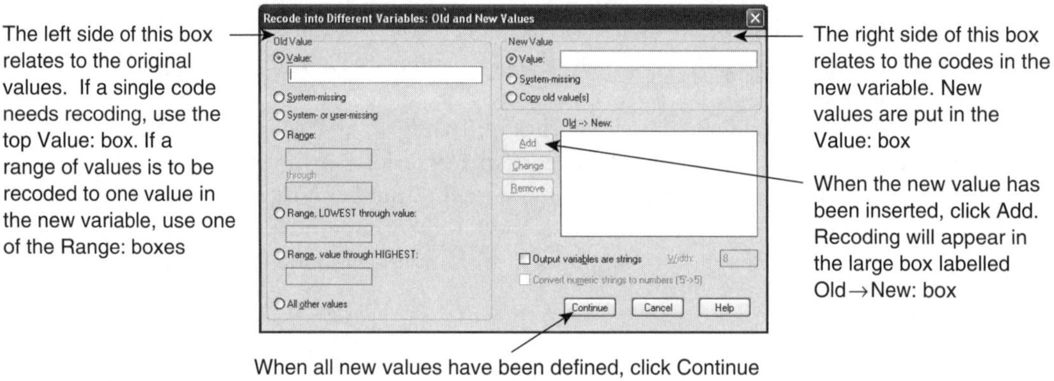

The left side of this box
relates to the original
values. If a single code
needs recoding, use the
top Value: box. If a
range of values is to be
recoded to one value in
the new variable, use one
of the Range: boxes

The right side of this box
relates to the codes in the
new variable. New
values are put in the
Value: box

When the new value has
been inserted, click Add.
Recoding will appear in
the large box labelled
Old→New: box

When all new values have been defined, click Continue

FIGURE 2.3   RECODE INTO DIFFERENT VARIABLES: OLD AND NEW VALUES DIALOG BOX

once the variable has been defined) to label the new variable by filling in the Label:
box. When these have been completed, click the Change button and the new variable name will be transferred to the Input Variable → Output Variable: box. Next
click Old and New Values… to give a dialog box like the one in Figure 2.3.

Looking at Figure 2.1, the aim of this recoding is to code the three white ethnicities together, the black ethnicities plus mixed black and white together and finally
all other categories together, so that there are three categories ('white', 'black' and
'other'). Missing data in the original variable will remain missing with the new variable. To recode a variable, it will probably be necessary to refer to Variable View so
that the right numerical codes are recoded. In the ethnicity example, the three white
ethnicities are coded 1, 2 and 3; with the new variable they will be recoded to 1. On
the left hand side of the dialog box (under Old Value) in Figure 2.3, click on the first
Range: radio button to activate the boxes below; put 1 in the top box and 3 in the
box below 'through'. On the right hand side of the dialog box (under New Value),
in the Value box put 1. Then click Add. The changes that will occur will then be

Ethnic group

		Frequency	Percent	Valid Percent	Cumulative Percent
Valid	white	65	40.1	41.4	41.4
	black	52	32.1	33.1	74.5
	other	40	24.7	25.5	100.0
	Total	157	96.9	100.0	
Missing	System	5	3.1		
Total		162	100.0		

FIGURE 2.4   ETHNICITY VARIABLE FOLLOWING RECODING

Note: the value labels were defined using Variable View before Figure 2.4 was produced.

shown in the large white box on the right hand side of the dialog box, headed Old → New:. The 'black' and 'other' groups are recoded in a similar way. When all coding has been declared then press Continue, to return to the Recode into Different Variables dialog box (Figure 2.2). On that dialog box click OK. New variables are placed at the far right of the dataset in Data View, and at the bottom of the variable list in Variable View. The attributes of the variable can be altered in Variable View once the variable has been created in the same way as setting up a datasheet for data entry (Chapter 1). For example, for a categorical variable, it may be beneficial to define the Values as well as change the Measure (the default is Scale).

To make sure the recoding carried out produced the expected results, it is advisable to compare the frequencies of the new variable with the old variable (Figure 2.1). For the new variable, the frequency table shows 65 of 157 (41%) women were white, 52 (33%) were black and 40 (26%) were other ethnicity (Figure 2.4). As there should be, there are the same number of missing values in the original coding (Figure 2.1) of ethnicity and the recoded variable (Figure 2.4).

As the Recode into Different Variables: Old and New Values dialog box (Figure 2.3) shows, there are a number of options about how to specify the old values depending on how the original variable was coded in relation to how the new variable is to be coded. For example, if the aim was to change the coding of a variable for logistic regression from 1 and 2 to 1 and 0 (recoding 2 to 0) then 2 would be placed in the Value: box under Old Value and 0 placed in the Value: box under New Value. As previously the Add button has to be clicked to register the changes. Changes are only made when the Continue button has been clicked on the Recode into Different Variables: Old and New Values dialog box (Figure 2.3), followed by OK on the Recode into Different Variables dialog box (Figure 2.2).

Another method that could have been used to define some of the old values of ethnicities in the student breast cancer awareness study is to define the values in terms as Range, LOWEST through value: since the white group was coded 1, 2 and 3; and there were no codes below one, 3 could have been placed in the box next to Range, LOWEST through value: and as before 1 placed in the Value: box on the New Value side of the dialog box (Figure 2.5). A similar principle applies for the Range, value through HIGHEST: box.

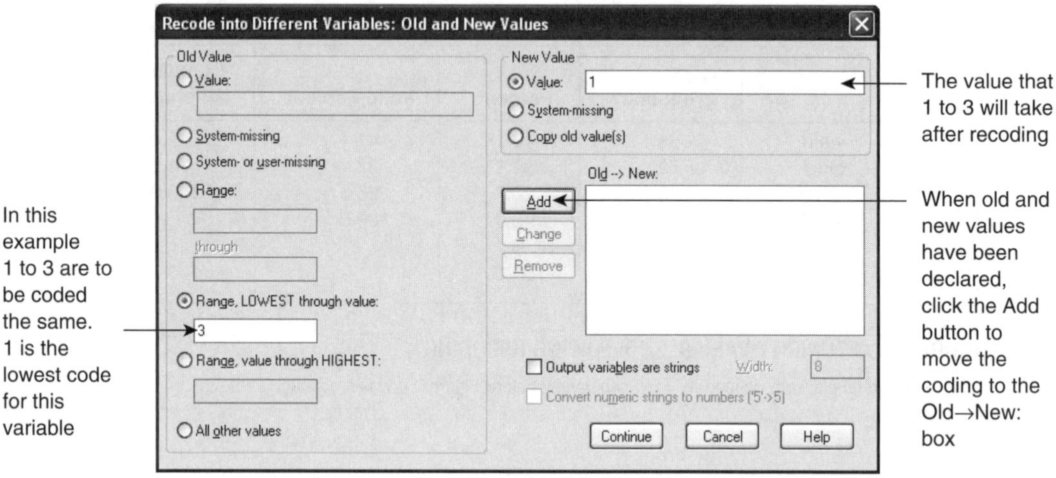

FIGURE 2.5   RECODE INTO DIFFERENT VARIABLES: OLD AND NEW VALUES, EXAMPLE OF LOWEST THROUGH VALUE

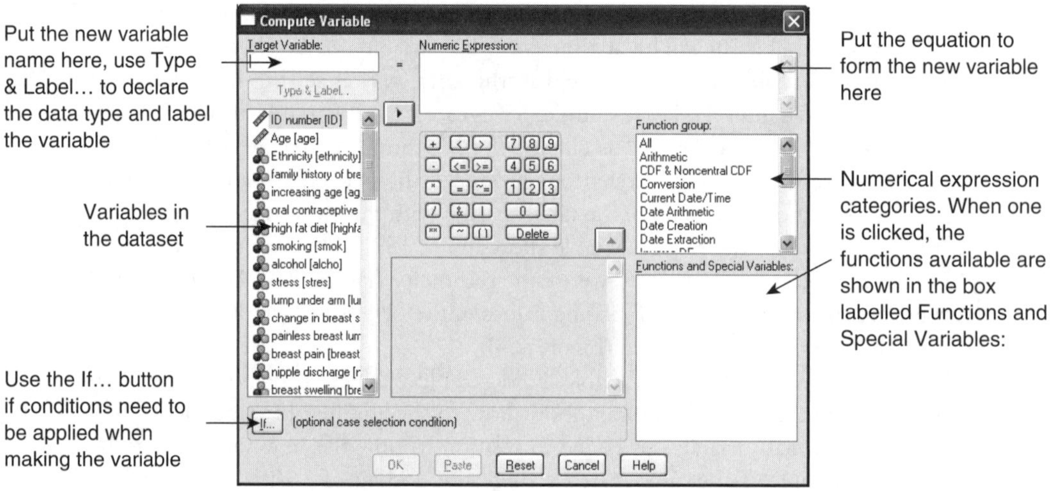

FIGURE 2.6   COMPUTE VARIABLE DIALOG BOX

CREATING NEW VARIABLES

It is often necessary to create new variables. This may be to create dummy variables for linear regression analysis (explained in Chapter 11); to combine data from more than one related variables to create a new variable or to manipulate the data using a function such as natural logarithms.

Whatever the reason for creating a new variable, the procedure starts by clicking on Transform → Compute Variable... to give the Compute Variable dialog box (Figure 2.6). Into the Target Variable: box, type the new variable name. Once a variable name has been added, the Type & Label... button becomes functional. This can be used to declare the type of data and to label the variable. Both of these can also be declared or edited in Variable View after the variable has been computed.

The first example of computing variables shown will be to create dummy variables which can then be used as independent variables in linear regression. Linear regression is explained further in Chapter 11.

Dummy (indicator) variables

Where a categorical variable has more than two categories, the user has to make dummy (sometimes referred to as indicator) variables so that a linear regression coefficient can be calculated for each category within a variable. Dummy variables are a series of mutually exclusive dichotomous variables that represent all categories within the original variable. These are usually coded 0 indicating without the characteristic in question and 1 indicating with the variable in question. This textual example will use categorical age data from the obesity dataset (as this variable is used in multiple linear regression in Chapter 11).

In the original variable 1 = less than 20 years, 2 = 20 to 30 years, 3 = 31 to 40 years, 4 = 41 to 50 years and 5 = 51 to 60 years. There were no participants aged less than 20 years in the dataset. When constructing dummy variables, one category has to be designated the reference category, that is, the one which the other categories are compared to. In the example shown in Table 2.1 category 2 (age 20 to 30 years) will be the reference category. This means that it will not be necessary to create a variable representing this age group. For the other age categories, it is necessary to create new variables that equal 0 if the participant is not a member of the age category in question and 1 if they are. For example, looking at Table 2.1, the original coding of the variable is shown in the Age category column, with the following three columns being the dummy variables (Age31–40 representing age 31 to 40, Age41–50 representing age 41 to 50 and Age5160 representing age 51 to 60. Looking at the variable Age31–40, the only occasions where it takes 1 is where the value in the Age category variable is 3 (indicating 31 to 40 years in the original variable). Likewise, this is repeated in Age41–50 and Age51–60, with these variables taking 1 where Age category equals 4 and 5 respectively. Dummy variables can be constructed by recoding into a different variable using SPSS.

TABLE 2.1   CODING OF DUMMY VARIABLES – AN EXTRACT FROM THE AGE CATEGORY FROM THE OBESITY DATASET

Age category	Age 31–40	Age 41–50	Age 51–60
2	0	0	0
4	0	1	0
2	0	0	0
2	0	0	0
2	0	0	0
2	0	0	0
2	0	0	0
3	1	0	0
4	0	1	0
3	1	0	0
5	0	0	1
2	0	0	0

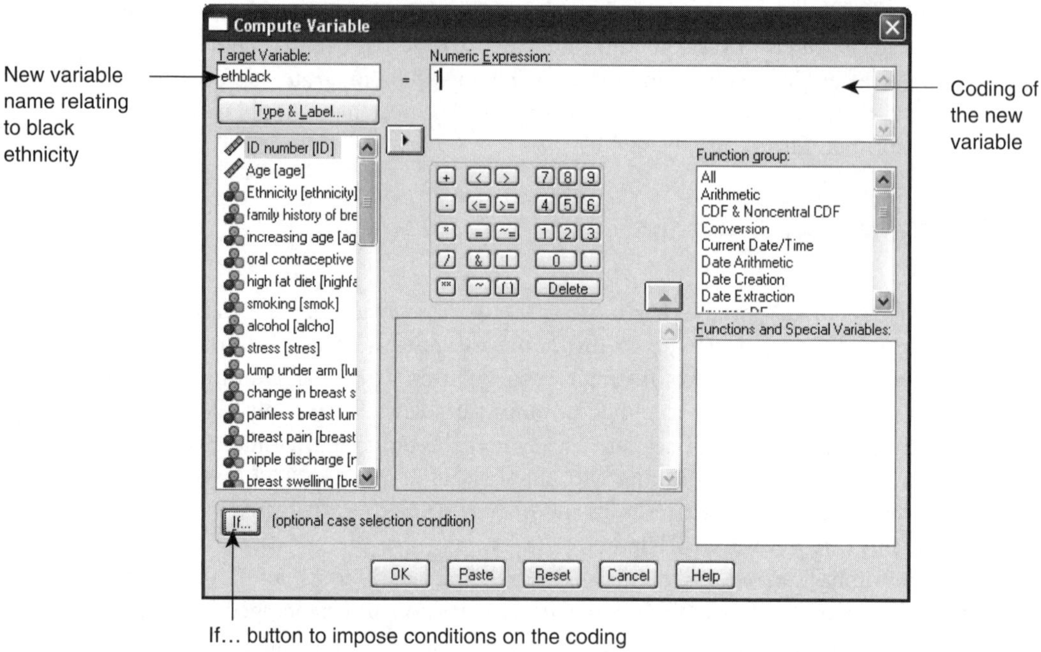

New variable name relating to black ethnicity

Coding of the new variable

If... button to impose conditions on the coding

FIGURE 2.7   COMPUTE VARIABLE DIALOG BOX TO CREATE DUMMY VARIABLES

Figure 2.7 shows the student breast cancer awareness dataset. The variable to be made into a dummy variable is ethnicity, which has already been recoded (from the large number of categories the data were collected in) to three categories (white, black and other) earlier in this chapter. Two variables need to be created: black versus not black and other ethnicity versus not other ethnicity. White will be the reference category, so that if a participant is coded as not black and not other ethnicity, then as long as there is not missing data for that participant they will be white. Figure 2.7 shows the target variable (new variable name) is ethblack; this variable will be the dummy relating to black ethnicity. 1 has been placed in the Numeric Expression: box as that will indicate that the participant is black. However, not all women in this study were black, the If... button should be clicked to give the Compute Variable: If Cases dialog box shown in Figure 2.8. This is used so that only the women who are black are coded 1 with the dummy variable. Therefore in the Compute Variable: If Cases dialog box (Figure 2.8), click the radio button next to Include if case satisfies condition: then in the white box at the top of the dialog box (Figure 2.8), put the original ethnicity variable = the required coding of the original variable. For example, Figure 2.8 shows ethgroup = 2 because black is coded 2 in that variable. When that has been completed click Continue to return to the Compute Variable dialog box (Figure 2.7), then click OK.

The new variable will be situated at the far right of the dataset. It contains values where the coding is 1 (corresponding to the black participants). To fill in the remainder of the variable (where there is information on ethnicity, but the participant is not black) to 0 click on Transform → Recode into Same Variables... to give the Recode into Same Variables dialog box as shown in Figure 2.9. Move the variable to be recoded to the Numeric Variables: box. In this example, this is ethblack. Then click on

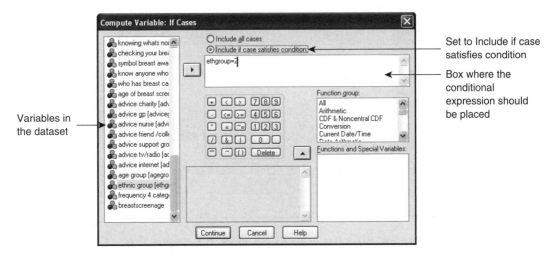

Variables in
the dataset

Set to Include if case
satisfies condition

Box where the
conditional
expression should
be placed

FIGURE 2.8   COMPUTE VARIABLE: IF CASES DIALOG BOX

If… to give the Recode into Same Variables: If Cases dialog box (Figure 2.10). Within
this, a condition to only include those participants where there is not missing data in
the original variable will be set up. Therefore change the radio button to select
Include if case satisfies condition:, then enter the appropriate expression in the large
white box (in Figure 2.10 this equates to the variable ethgroup not having missing
data). When the expression has been entered click Continue to return to the Recode
into Same Variables dialog box (Figure 2.9). The condition constructed will then
appear next to the If… button, where (optional case selection condition) is shown in
Figure 2.9. Then click on the Old and New Values… button to give the Recode into
Same Variables: Old and New Values dialog box (Figure 2.11). On the Old Value side
of the dialog box selected the System-Missing radio button and on the new values
side of the dialog box put 0 in the Value: box. Then click Add followed by Continue
to return to the Recode into Same Variables dialog box (Figure 2.9), and finally click
OK. It is good practice to compare the frequencies of the original variable with the

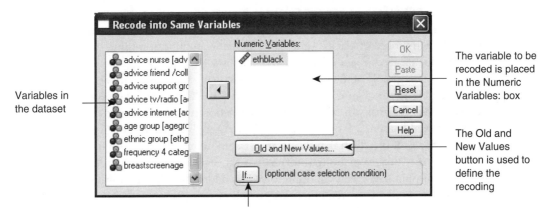

Variables in
the dataset

The variable to be
recoded is placed
in the Numeric
Variables: box

The Old and
New Values
button is used to
define the
recoding

Use the If… button to set conditions for recoding given cases

FIGURE 2.9   RECODE INTO SAME VARIABLES DIALOG BOX

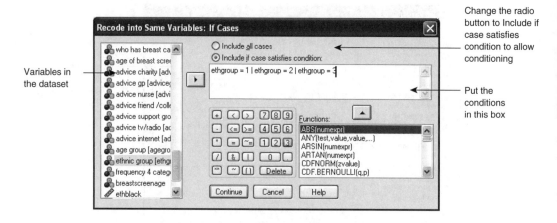

FIGURE 2.10   RECODE INTO SAME VARIABLES: IF CASES DIALOG BOX

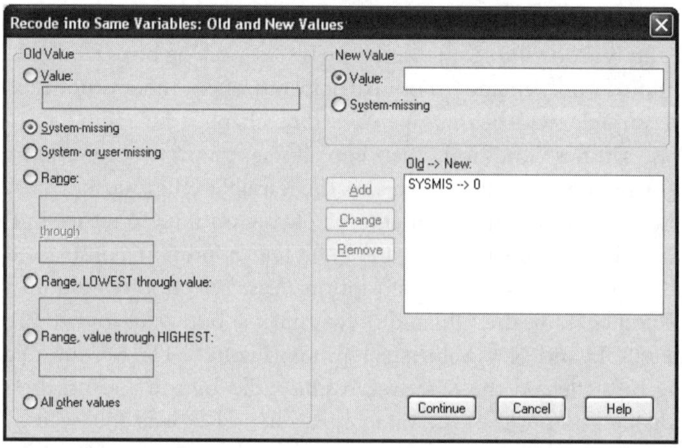

FIGURE 2.11   RECODE INTO SAME VARIABLES: OLD AND NEW VALUES DIALOG BOX

new variable to make sure the new variable is giving the same frequencies (in terms of missing and present data). These are shown in Figure 2.12; where the new variable has the same number of black women and the same amount of missing data. As previously value labels can be declared in Variable View.

The second example of the use of Compute Variable is to create a variable containing the natural logarithm of an existing continuous variable. This may be necessary when a variable is not Normally distributed as transformation can (but does not always) normalise skewed variables. However, it should be noted that if the original variable includes values of 0 (which may occur in variables representing health or quality of life scales), 0 is unable to be transformed to the natural logarithm scale (it would appear as missing data). This can be resolved by adding a small amount (0.5 or less) to each observation then remembering to subtract the amount added when back transforming for interpretation purposes.

If a skewed variable is transformed it may be possible to use parametric methods for analysis. Figure 2.13 shows a histogram of BMI from the student obesity dataset;

Ethnic black

		Frequency	Percent	Valid Percent	Cumulative Percent
Valid	0	105	64.8	66.9	66.9
	1	52	32.1	33.1	100.0
	Total	157	96.9	100.0	
Missing	System	5	3.1		
Total		162	100.0		

Ethnic group

		Frequency	Percent	Valid Percent	Cumulative Percent
Valid	White	65	40.1	41.4	41.4
	Black	52	32.1	33.1	74.5
	Other	40	24.7	25.5	100.0
	Total	157	96.9	100.0	
Missing	System	5	3.1		
Total		162	100.0		

FIGURE 2.12   FREQUENCIES OF THE BLACK ETHNIC VARIABLE AND ETHNIC GROUP VARIABLE

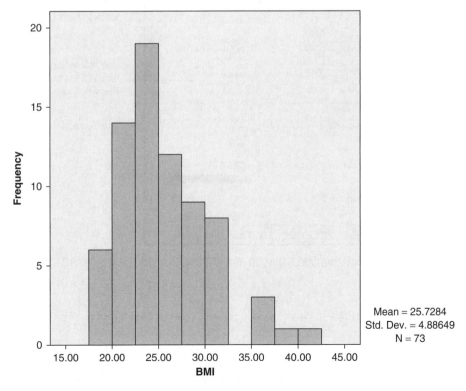

Mean = 25.7284
Std. Dev. = 4.88649
N = 73

FIGURE 2.13   HISTOGRAM OF BMI FROM THE STUDENT OBESITY DATASET

it shows BMI is a little right skewed with more observations towards the lower end of the range with a small number of participants with a BMI of 35 or more. The mean BMI is 25.7 (SD 4.9). As the skew is not severe in this variable, it would be at the discretion of the user (and also considering whether the assumptions of statistical tests had been met) whether to transform this variable.

As with the previous example the new variable name has to be defined by completing the Target Variable: box (Figure 2.14) in the Compute Variable dialog box before variables and functions can be added to the Numeric Expression: box. Then select the LN function from the Functions and Special Variables: list from the Compute Variable dialog box and transfer it to the Numeric Expression: box using the upward pointing arrow. The insertion point should be between the brackets (if not, it should be moved to between the brackets); this is where the existing variable should be transferred from the variable list so that the Compute Variable dialog box appears like the one shown in Figure 2.14. When this has been completed click OK; the new variable has been created and will be situated at the right of the dataset. The distribution of the new variable is shown in Figure 2.15. This can be seen to be more Normally distributed than the original variable (Figure 2.13).

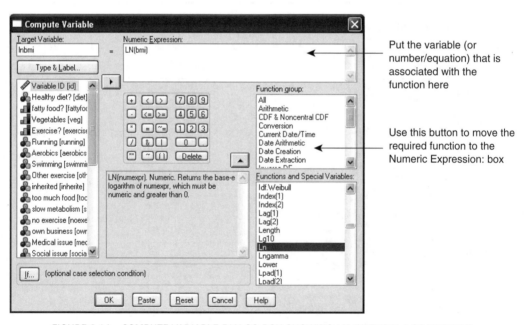

FIGURE 2.14   COMPUTE VARIABLE DIALOG BOX SHOWING LN (NATURAL LOGARITHMS) EXAMPLE

SELECTING CASES

Sometimes it may be necessary to exclude some data on the basis of the responses to a particular variable. For example, there may an interest in characteristics of one gender or ethnicity only.

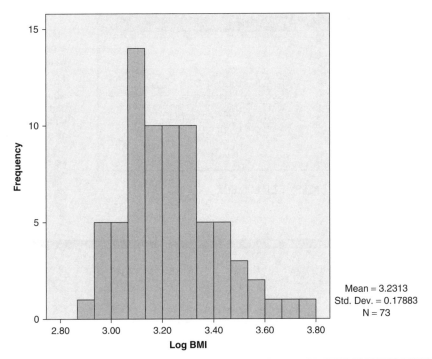

FIGURE 2.15   HISTOGRAM OF THE LOGARITHM OF BMI FROM THE STUDENT OBESITY DATASET

Click on Data → Select cases… . The Select Cases dialog box (Figure 2.16) will appear. To only use cases with specific characteristics, click on the If condition is satisfied radio button, then click the If… button to get the Select Cases: If dialog box (Figure 2.17). In this dialog box, the algorithm representing the condition should be

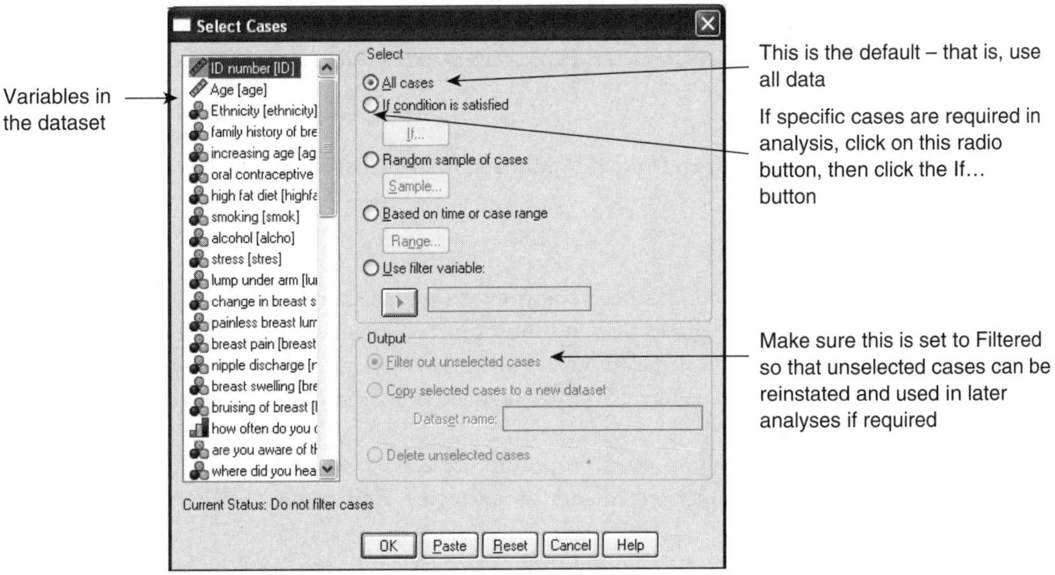

FIGURE 2.16   SELECT CASES DIALOG BOX

Variables in the dataset →

The function which constitutes the cases wanted is put here →

Numerical, arithmetic and logical function buttons. These can also be accessed using the computer keyboard

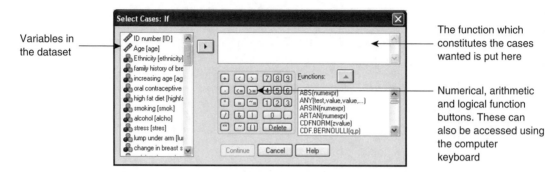

FIGURE 2.17   SELECT CASES: IF DIALOG BOX

In Data View, cases that are not being used are denoted with a diagonal line through the number →

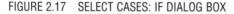

This indicates that cases are being filtered out

FIGURE 2.18   SCREENSHOT SHOWING HOW NON-SELECTED CASES ARE INDICATED IN DATA VIEW

placed. When the condition has been constructed (in the example shown in Figure 2.18 this is to select cases if ethgroup=1 in the breast cancer awareness dataset), click Continue, to return to the Select Cases dialog box (Figure 2.16) then click OK. In Figure 2.18 the observations that have been filtered out are signified by a diagonal line through the SPSS numerical identifier.

In addition, the selecting cases procedure creates a new variable filter_$, which takes the values 0 for not selected and 1 for selected. This is shown in Variable View (Figure 2.19).

When the whole dataset is required after using Select Cases, from the Select Cases dialog box (Figure 2.16) select the All cases radio button then click OK.

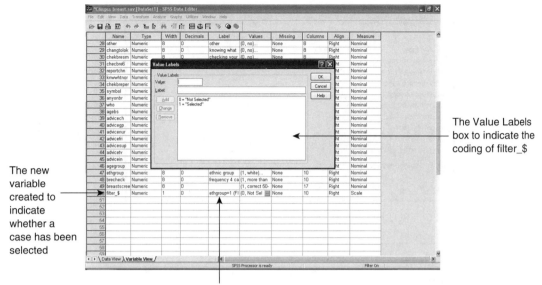

The new variable created to indicate whether a case has been selected

The Value Labels box to indicate the coding of filter_$

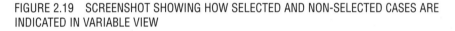

The Label indicates the filtering criteria

FIGURE 2.19   SCREENSHOT SHOWING HOW SELECTED AND NON-SELECTED CASES ARE INDICATED IN VARIABLE VIEW

SPLIT FILE

This is used if statistics are required separately by a given variable. For example, you might want to look at characteristics of members of a dataset by social class or age group. Summary statistics and other analyses can then be carried out on each defined group.

To split a file click on Data → Split File... to get the Split File dialog box shown in Figure 2.20. Select the radio button Organize output by groups. One or more variables in the dataset then have to be transferred to the Groups Based on: box. When this has been done, click OK. There will be no indicators that the file has been split when looking at the dataset in Data View or Variable View. It will only be apparent when data are analysed. For example, in Figure 2.21, the student breast cancer awareness data has been split by ethnic group then frequencies are shown for the variable 'Is increasing age a risk factor for breast cancer?' Frequencies for categorical data are explained further in Chapter 6.

Interpretation

The first set of statistics is for the group where ethnicity is missing (5 participants) and would not usually be reported. Following that it can be seen that 22% of white women thought increasing age was a risk factor for breast cancer and likewise 23% for black women and 13% for women from other ethnic groups.

To reverse splitting the file (so that all data are used again) click on Data → Split File... and select the radio button Analyze all cases, do not create groups, then click OK.

Variables in the dataset →

Make sure this radio button is selected

Move the variable(s) that you want to split the file by into this box

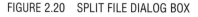

FIGURE 2.20   SPLIT FILE DIALOG BOX

ethnic group = .

Statistics[a]

increasing age

N	Valid	5
	Missing	0

[a]ethnic group =

increasing age[a]

		Frequency	Percent	Valid Percent	Cumulative Percent
Valid	no	3	60.0	60.0	60.0
	yes	2	40.0	40.0	100.0
	Total	5	100.0	100.0	

[a]ethnic group =

ethnic group = white

Statistics[a]

increasing age

N	Valid	65
	Missing	0

[a]ethnic group = white

increasing age[a]

		Frequency	Percent	Valid Percent	Cumulative Percent
Valid	no	51	78.5	78.5	78.5
	yes	14	21.5	21.5	100.0
	Total	65	100.0	100.0	

[a]ethnic group = white

FIGURE 2.21   (*Continued*)

ethnic group = black

Statistics[a]

increasing age[a]

N	Valid	52
	Missing	0

[a]ethnic group = black

increasing age[a]

		Frequency	Percent	Valid Percent	Cumulative Percent
Valid	no	40	76.9	76.9	76.9
	yes	12	23.1	23.1	100.0
	Total	52	100.0	100.0	

[a]ethnic group = black

ethnic group = other

Statistics[a]

increasing age

N	Valid	40
	Missing	0

[a]ethnic group = other

increasing age[a]

		Frequency	Percent	Valid Percent	Cumulative Percent
Valid	no	35	87.5	87.5	87.5
	yes	5	12.5	12.5	100.0
	Total	40	100.0	100.0	

[a]ethnic group = other

FIGURE 2.21   'IS INCREASING AGE A RISK FACTOR FOR BREAST CANCER?' BY ETHNIC GROUP AFTER SPLITTING THE FILE

SORTING DATA

Sometimes it is necessary for a given variable to be in numerical order, either ascending or descending. This may be to find an extreme value within a variable so that it can be checked or because merging to add variables requires the variable to be matched on to be sorted in ascending order. This is illustrated with the student breast cancer awareness study. To sort data in SPSS click on Data → Sort Cases… to give the Sort Cases dialog box shown in Figure 2.22. The variable(s) that are to be

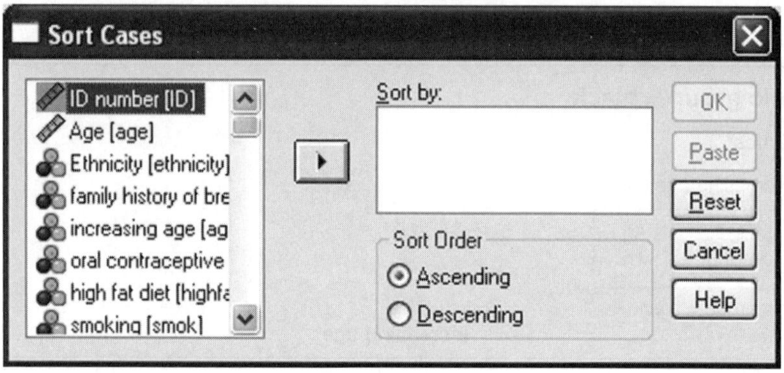

FIGURE 2.22   SORT CASES DIALOG BOX

merge, it is likely that the merge will be on ID number, so this would be transferred to the Sort by: box. When the sort by variables and their ordering has been declared, click OK to return to the sorted dataset.

MERGING

This is useful when there are two datasets containing either the same variables or the same participants, and their information needs to be combined to make one dataset for analysis purposes. For example, data may be collected at more than one time point, often analysis uses data collected at both (all) time points. This occurs when longitudinal datasets, such as the Millennium Cohort Study are being analysed, whereby data are supplied in files according to the time period they were collected in. The case where additional participants are added to a dataset occurs less frequently, but may occur when colleagues have been collecting the same data from different participants and have recorded it in different SPSS datasets, which need to be merged before analysis can take place.

The case where new variables are added is to be explored first. This example will use the student breast cancer awareness data. For this example the dataset has been bisected with most variables in one dataset and a few additional ones in another dataset. Before beginning the merge process, make sure that both datasets are sorted in ascending order on the variable which links the two datasets (in this dataset it is the ID number) otherwise the merge will not be executed. To execute a merge of datasets in SPSS to add variables, with the main dataset open, click on Data → Merge Files → Add Variables… to get the Add Variables to [open dataset] dialog box shown in Figure 2.23.

When a second dataset containing the additional variables has been selected, either through the datasets open or through browsing; click Continue to go to the Add Variables from [second dataset] dialog box (Figure 2.24). In this box, the majority of variables appear in the New Active Dataset: box, showing which variables will appear in the new dataset. Any variables that appear in both datasets (with exactly the same variable name) will be in the Excluded Variables: box. In this example this applies to ID. However, this variable is not to be excluded as this is the variable that is used to

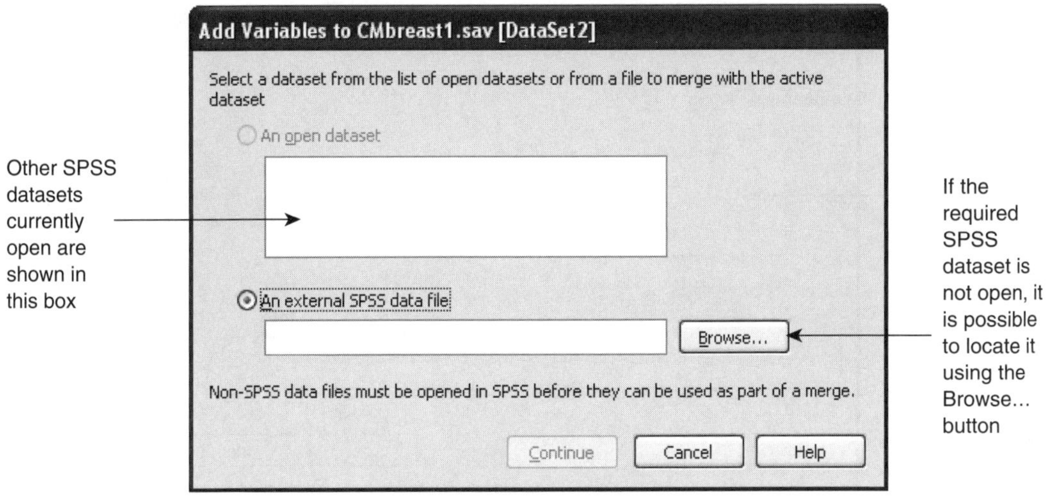

Other SPSS datasets currently open are shown in this box

If the required SPSS dataset is not open, it is possible to locate it using the Browse... button

FIGURE 2.23   ADD VARIABLES TO [OPEN DATASET] DIALOG BOX

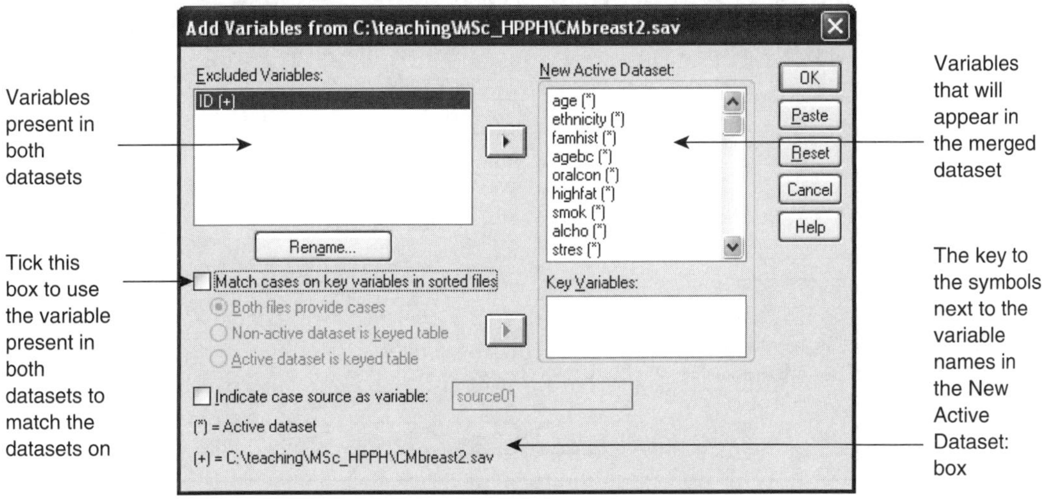

Variables present in both datasets

Tick this box to use the variable present in both datasets to match the datasets on

Variables that will appear in the merged dataset

The key to the symbols next to the variable names in the New Active Dataset: box

FIGURE 2.24   ADD VARIABLES FROM [SECOND DATASET] DIALOG BOX

match data from the two datasets; so that it can be ensured that data from participants in one dataset are from the same participants in the other dataset. For this to happen, the Match cases on key variables in sorted files box should be ticked, then ensuring the Both files provide cases radio button is selected (this is the default), then move the variable from the Excluded Variables: box to the Key Variables: box. Then click OK. The merge will then be complete and variables from both datasets will be visible in the first dataset. This should be saved so that the results of merging are not lost.

The second possible situation covered by merging is where data from additional participants is added to the main dataset. This is also going to be explained using the student breast cancer awareness study; this time the dataset is bisected horizontally so

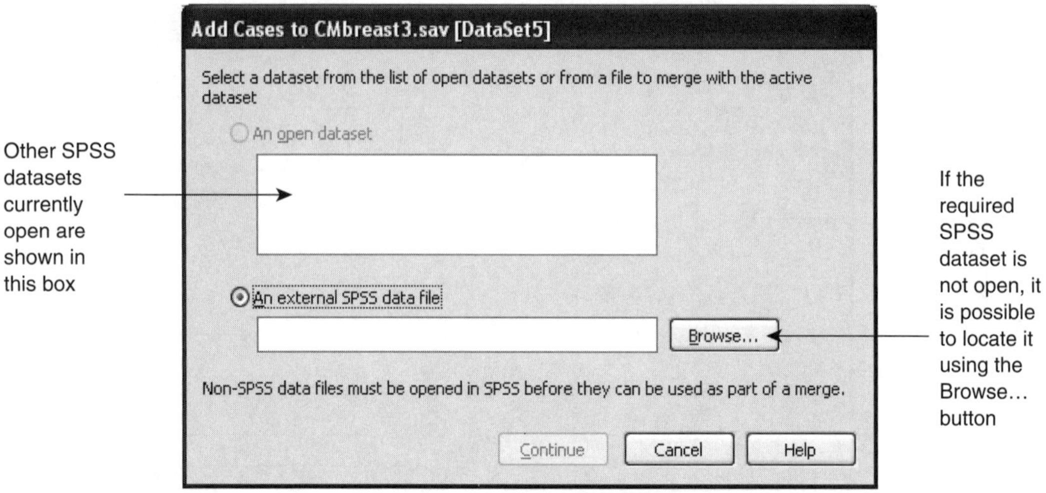

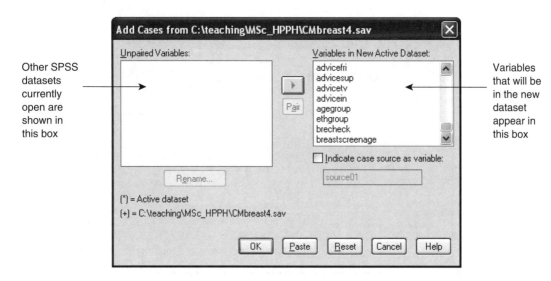

Other SPSS datasets currently open are shown in this box

If the required SPSS dataset is not open, it is possible to locate it using the Browse... button

FIGURE 2.25   ADD CASES TO [OPEN DATASET] DIALOG BOX

Other SPSS datasets currently open are shown in this box

Variables that will be in the new dataset appear in this box

FIGURE 2.26   ADD CASES FROM [SECOND DATASET] DIALOG BOX

that the main dataset contains 100 participants whilst the second dataset contains the remainder of the participants. In SPSS, this merge is invoked by clicking on Data → Merge Files → Add Cases... when the main dataset is open to get the Add Cases to [open dataset] dialog box (Figure 2.25). The aim of this dialog box is to locate the dataset to be merged into the open dataset; this can either be a dataset that is already open (these will be shown in the An open dataset box), or a dataset that is not open, which can be searched for using the Browse... button.

When the dataset has been selected, click Continue to give the Add Cases from [second dataset] dialog box (Figure 2.26). The aim of this dialog box is show the variables that will be in the new dataset (in the Variables in New Active Dataset: box) and where necessary pair variables with different variable names which are representing the same variable (shown in the Unpaired Variables: box). In the example shown in Figure 2.26 there are no variables where this is the case. When any unpaired variable issues have been resolved, click OK to give the complete dataset. Remember to save the new dataset.

SUMMARY

- Sometimes it is necessary to recode variables for analysis. To do this, click on Transform → Recode into different variables….
- New variables can be computed using Transform → Compute Variable ….
- Cases can be selected on the basis of variable(s) in the dataset using Data → Select Cases….
- The file can be split so that further analysis can be carried out by given variable(s), using Data → Split file….
- Variables within a dataset can be sorted in either ascending or descending order by clicking on Data → Sort Cases….
- Datasets can be merged so that either more variables are added or more cases (participants or subjects) are added. This can be done using Data → Merge Files.

EXERCISES

Open obesity.sav:

1 Recode the variable 'agegroup' into the same variable so that 0 = those aged 11 to 30 years, 1 = those aged 31 to 40 years and 2 = those aged 41+ years. Remember to change the value labels when the recoding is complete.
2 Make a new variable using BMI to produce a dichotomous variable indicating obese (BMI 30+) versus not obese. Remember to consider missing data.
3 Create dummy variables for the variable 'exercise'. Use 'never' as the reference category.
4 Sort the dataset to find the largest and smallest BMI.

3
STUDY DESIGNS

INTRODUCTION

Whether carried out by students to fulfil their degree requirements or researchers and health professionals, all research studies have to be planned and the study designed in such a way that it answers the research questions. Research studies can be observational or experimental. Observational studies are those where the researcher aims to discover what conditions the participants have, their measurements and/or their opinions. None of the conditions experienced by the participants are manipulated by the researchers. This contrasts with experimental studies where many conditions are controlled by the researchers.

This chapter will describe four main types of study design which are commonly used within the healthcare setting. These are cross sectional studies, case–control studies, cohort studies and randomised controlled trials, the first three being observational and the latter being experimental.

THE AIMS OF THIS CHAPTER ARE:

- To know the appropriate study design for the research questions being asked.
- To describe features of commonly used study designs.

CROSS SECTIONAL STUDIES

Cross sectional studies are the most common for student projects because they are relatively quick and cheap to undertake for the researcher. This is because they involve a single group of participants at one time point, often using surveys (question-naires). Therefore the researcher does not have to make contact with participants on multiple occasions to gain data from them. Student projects often use convenience sampling for their cross sectional studies. Convenience sampling is explained further in Chapter 7.

In cross sectional studies data can be collected about the past, but no data were collected prior to the encounter with the researcher. If questions that rely on memory are used, then there is the possibility of data being subject to recall bias. This is where participants misrecall events from the past; giving incorrect data. Additionally, as data are collected at one time point, this means that the outcome and exposure data are collected at the same time. This has the disadvantage of it being unclear which came about first. For example, questions on cancer status are asked at the same time as smoking status so it is unclear which came first and to what degree they affected one another.

Cross sectional studies can also be prevalence studies which aim to discover the prevalence of a disease, condition or event in a sample of representative participants. If inferences are to be made from prevalence studies, then it is important that the sample is representative of the relevant population.

The data collected could be descriptive or analytical. Descriptive studies look at characteristics, opinions and/or continuous measurements (such as blood pressure) to give a picture of the participants in the context that they are included in the study. Analytical studies are used to elicit associations between factors and/or identify risk factors for a given disease, event or condition. Analytical cross sectional studies utilise descriptive statistics before moving onto further inferential analysis.

Example from the literature

Objective: To determine if risky sexual intercourse, sexually transmitted diseases, and sexual intercourse at an early age are associated with psychiatric disorder.

Design: Cross sectional study of a birth cohort at age 21 years with assessments presented by computer (for sexual behaviour) and by trained interviewers (for psychiatric disorder).

Setting: New Zealand in 1993–4.

Participants: 992 study members (487 women) from the Dunedin multidisciplinary health and development study. Complete data were available on both measures for 930 study members.

Main outcome measures: Psychiatric disorders (anxiety, depression, eating disorder, substance dependence, antisocial disorder, mania, schizophrenia spectrum) and measures of sexual behaviour.

Results: Young people diagnosed with substance dependence, schizophrenia spectrum, and antisocial disorders were more likely to engage in risky sexual intercourse, contract sexually transmitted diseases, and have sexual intercourse at an early age (before 16 years). Unexpectedly, so were young people with depressive disorders. Young people with mania were more likely to report risky sexual intercourse and have sexually transmitted diseases. The likelihood of risky behaviour was increased by psychiatric comorbidity.

Conclusions: There is a clear association between risky sexual behaviour and common psychiatric disorders. Although the temporal relation is uncertain, the results indicate the need to coordinate sexual medicine with mental health services in the treatment of young people. (Ramrakha et al., 2000: 263)

The Objective given in Ramrakha et al.'s (2000) abstract indicates that the study is analytical because possible relationships between psychiatric disorders and sexual behaviour were examined. The Design indicates that data on psychiatric disorders and sexual behaviour were collected at the same time, which is reflected in the Conclusions where the authors state '*Although the temporal relation is uncertain…*' (my emphasis) indicating they do not know whether psychiatric disorders or sexual behaviours came first.

Large scale data collection sometimes uses cross sectional study design. For example, in England, the Health Survey for England is completed annually asking a large battery of questions and collecting some physical measurements from members of a random sample of households in England. A core set of questions are asked every year, with questions pertaining to particular themes being included each year. Therefore, trends over time can be examined by analysing successive surveys, but the respondents cannot be followed over time to determine whether and/or when respondents get a disease or condition or experience a given event because a different random sample is selected annually.

Example from the literature

The Health Survey for England is an annual survey of people living in private households in England conducted by the National Centre for Social Surveys and Research and University College London on behalf of the Department of Health. The 1999 survey focused on the health of minority ethnic groups.

Three separate samples were obtained. Firstly, a general population sample of 6552 households was obtained using two-stage random sampling of postcode sectors and then addresses within each sector. Second, an 'ethnic boost' sample of 26 528 addresses was obtained using stratified multistage probability sampling. Additional postcode sectors were selected as primary sampling units. The sampling of postcode sectors was systematic to include a greater proportion from areas with a high percentage of minority ethnic groups. Each household in the ethnic boost sample was screened initially and only included if respondents identified themselves as belonging to an ethnic minority group. A third sample was obtained for Chinese informants by following up 569 households who took part in a Health Education Authority survey in 1998. All participating households were interviewed in full. (Saxena et al., 2004: 30)

The paper by Saxena et al. (2004) used data from the Health Survey for England 1999, mainly because they were examining ethnic differences in overweight and obesity in young people in England. In 1999 minority ethnic groups were over-sampled. It would have been difficult to have looked at such differences if minority ethnic groups had not been oversampled because only 9% of the population of England is from a minority ethnic group (ONS, 2001) and using data from the normal population composition of England would have meant that the numbers in each ethnic group would have been too small to make meaningful inferences. The methods section of this paper continues by explaining how the sample was achieved.

CASE-CONTROL STUDIES

Case-control studies are usually retrospective, so that a current disease or condition is related to past exposures. They are used to answer questions of the form: 'Do persons with a disease or condition have a characteristic more frequently than those without the disease or condition?'

They involve taking a group of participants who have the condition or disease of interest and a group who do not have the condition or disease. These are known as the cases and controls respectively. Information is then collected on possible exposures and causative factors to determine whether there are differences in exposure status between the two groups. As case-control studies start with the cases and looks back to possible causative factors, they are good for rare diseases or conditions.

Cases are usually identified in one of two ways: from disease registries, for example cancer registries; or by a process of referral and investigation, for example, patients in a given hospital with the disease or condition in question may be referred to the study coordinators. At this point, they decide whether potential cases fit the inclusion criteria, which should be well defined in terms of the disease or condition as well as other possible criteria such as age or quality of documentation of the disease or condition. It is often better to recruit incident (newly diagnosed) cases to the study because they are likely to have better recall of prior exposures than people who were diagnosed some time previously.

The controls should be selected with care so that they are comparable with the cases apart from not having the condition or disease of interest. Ideally, they should be selected from the same source as the cases. However, there are caveats to that: for example if cases are participants with breast cancer recruited from a hospital out-patient clinic, it is not advisable to recruit controls from another oncology clinic because of the possible interrelationships between cancers and their risk factors (for example, smoking status). It would be possible to recruit from another out-patient clinic, unrelated to oncology in the hospital. In this example, controls should not be male, since participants to this study would be exclusively female.

Sometimes controls are matched to cases using one or more baseline characteristic such as age, sex or geographical location. This ensures that baseline characteristics are the same between cases and controls and therefore these characteristics do not need to be controlled for in analysis. It can be difficult to match on a number of factors because it can be hard to find participants who fit the criteria for matching properly.

It is important not to over match cases and controls; that is, matching on too many factors. If cases and controls are matched on a factor related to exposure, then there is an increased chance that cases and controls will have the same exposure history and it would therefore be more difficult to determine factors associated with the disease or condition in question.

Some studies have more than one control per case. Often these controls are taken from different sources; so one control may be taken from the hospital that the cases are recruited from whilst the second control may be recruited from the community, possibly GP practices close to where the cases live.

Case-control studies are analysed using odds ratios. These will be discussed further in Chapter 12.

Example from the literature

> The aim of the study was to examine the null hypothesis that a used infant mattress is not associated with an increased risk of sudden infant death syndrome.
>
> The Registrar General for Scotland reported to us all infant deaths occurring after the seventh day of life to the end of the first year and provided the computerised maternity record. For sudden unexpected deaths, we were notified directly by the pathologist. A standard necropsy protocol with agreed diagnostic criteria was used to ensure consistent classification. We scrutinised all infant deaths for misclassification. Overall, 195 out of 751 postperinatal infant deaths were categorised as due to the sudden infant death syndrome between January 1996 and May 2000.
>
> We identified babies born immediately before and after the index case in the same maternity unit to act as controls. Controls were therefore matched for age, season, and maternity unit. We made home visits to complete a questionnaire within 28 days of the index case's death to minimise differences in age related circumstances between cases and controls. Questionnaires were completed on 131 of 195 cases and 278 controls. We were unable to acquire data on 64 cases because a delay in notification by the pathologist made it impossible to visit within 28 days of the death. The characteristics of the cases with and without an interview were similar in terms of maternal age and deprivation category. (Tappin et al., 2002)

The outcome in the paper by Tappin et al. (2002) was sudden infant death syndrome (SIDS). The study aimed to investigate whether there was a relationship between SIDS and whether the mattress had previously been used by another infant. The diagnosis was determined accurately as indicated by 'For sudden unexpected deaths, we were notified directly by the pathologist. A standard necropsy protocol with agreed diagnostic criteria was used to ensure consistent classification.' These were the cases. The paper also makes the source of the controls clear '…babies born immediately before and after the index case in the same maternity unit to act as controls.' As controls were selected from the birth register of the same maternity unit, and born at a similar time to the case, this meant that there was matching between cases and controls.

COHORT STUDIES

In cohort studies (sometimes called longitudinal studies), participants are selected for a common characteristic such as workplace or geography. The common characteristic could also be an experience such as being born prematurely, but should not be the outcome that the researchers are aiming to measure. If all participants had the outcome of interest it would be impossible to determine factors associated with it. Cohort studies can be carried out retrospectively using historical records to identify prospective participants and the occurrence of subsequent events. For example, such studies can be completed by linking a number of different types of routine records so that a picture of the health of a cohort can be constructed.

The majority of cohort studies are prospective. Prospective cohort studies can be conducted such that the participants are recruited to the study and are followed over time. The amount of time they are followed up for may be determined by the funding available for the study, a given number of years or until a predetermined event (such as death) occurs. The fact that this study design requires participants to provide information about themselves on a number of occasions implies that this study design is expensive for the researcher to carry out and that results may not be seen for a number of years. Data can be collected in a number of forms for example: structured interviews (which may give qualitative or quantitative data depending on the exact structure of the interview); questionnaires (for example, demographics, disease status, possible risk factors or health related quality of life instruments); records (these might be the routine medical records of individual participants or routine mortality or morbidity data); or physical examinations/tests. These may include the taking of blood for analysis and measuring weight and height.

Cohort studies have the disadvantage of possible bias over time. This is because as studies proceed, participants may become less interested in the research or cannot afford the time to take part in the study so the demographic and socioeconomic composition of the participants may change, meaning that the remaining cohort may not represent the population that it represented at the outset of the research. This may have implications for analysis and interpretation. Analysis may have to control for factors that changed between time points. Ways to do this will be discussed further in Chapters 11 and 12.

Cohort studies are used to answer questions of the form: 'Do persons with a given characteristic develop a disease more frequently than those who do not have the characteristic?' To be able to make correct inferences, all people with the common characteristic or a representative sample of such people needs to be involved in the study.

Information is collected on possible causative factors, such as smoking, exposure to chemicals and demographics. Cohort studies are good for situations where the exposure (possible causative factor) is rare, for example exposure to a chemical in a workplace environment. In this situation the characteristic of interest would be working with a given chemical, and recruitment would take place in workplaces that expose their employees to the chemical of interest. In prospective studies, once recruited, participants are followed over time, where further data are collected to discover whether they get the condition of interest. As none of the participants have the condition of interest at the outset of the study, the study design ensures that the exposure is measured before the condition of interest has been diagnosed. As cohort studies follow participants, often for years, they are inefficient for rare diseases or conditions because at the end of the study there will be very few participants with the condition of interest so, apart from being very expensive in terms of time and other resources (including money), the study would not provide useful inferences.

As participants do not have given diseases or conditions at the outset of the study, multiple outcomes can be investigated. For example, the primary outcome might be diagnosis of a specific type of cancer; however, secondary outcomes may be other types of cancer.

As cohort studies are representative of a population they are able to give a direct measure of incidence and prevalence within the study population and relative risks can be calculated. Relative risks will be shown in Chapter 8.

Example from the literature

Objectives: To identify risk factors for new episodes of sick leave due to neck or back pain.
Methods: This prospective study comprised an industrial population of 2187 employees who were followed up at 18 months and 3 years after a comprehensive baseline measurement. The potential risk factors comprised physical and psychosocial work factors, health-related and pain-related characteristics and lifestyle and demographic factors. The response rate at both follow-ups was close to 73%.
(Bergström et al., 2007: 279)

The Methods of this abstract indicates the study is going forward in time by using 'prospective'. This is further confirmed by the timing of follow-up being indicated by '…were followed up at 18 months and 3 years'. Returning to the Objectives, as they are 'To identify risk factors', this is an analytical study.

There are a number of ongoing large scale studies that are available in the UK Data Archive. These include the 1970 British Cohort Study and the Millennium Cohort Study. The 1970 British Cohort Study comprises people who were born in one particular week in 1970. Since birth there have been six data collection sweeps of the whole cohort at ages 5, 10, 16, 26, 29 and 34 years, with subsamples being collected at other times. The Millennium Cohort Study comprises a sample of approximately 19000 children born between September 2000 and August 2001. Since its inception, the Millennium Cohort Study has collected data at nine months, three years and five years with further data collection sweeps planned.

RANDOMISED CONTROLLED TRIALS (RCT)

Randomised controlled trials are considered to be the 'gold standard' of research designs. These are an experimental design whereby factors are controlled by the study coordinators so that it can be seen whether the intervention is more successful in treating the disease or condition in question than usual treatment. Randomised controlled trials have detailed protocols detailing the aims of the study, data analysis plans and procedures to be adhered to under given circumstances so all participants are treated in the same way. Randomised controlled trials are carried out because it is not known whether the intervention is more effective than usual treatment.

Randomised controlled trials are carried out by randomising participants to either the intervention or usual care (one of two groups). It is possible to design RCTs with more than two groups, but this chapter will focus on the case of two groups. Where there is no usual treatment in a drug trial, a placebo is used. This is inactive, but it is made to resemble the active drug in terms of look, consistency, smell and taste. Placebos can also take the form of saline injections or sham treatment (for example, acupuncture in insensitive areas). Placebos are used to discover whether the intervention is better than no treatment whilst minimising bias in the study. Where there are two groups in the trial, before entering the study, potential participants have a 50% probability of being randomised to each group.

Randomisation can be done using random number tables, computer programs or through a randomisation service. This ensures that allocation is not systematic, whereby it could be worked out what the next allocation is, and could therefore be open to abuse creating bias. Examples of allocations that are not random include assigning every other participant to the intervention, with others receiving usual care or allocating those with an even numbered month of birth to the intervention and those with an odd numbered month of birth to usual care. These allocation methods are open to abuse since it would be known in advance of allocation what an individual would be assigned to.

By randomising participants to their groups the baseline characteristics of the two groups should be similar and any differences would have occurred by chance. This means that any differences that are observed after treatment has been administered are likely to be due to the treatment.

Ideally randomised controlled trials should be double blind so that the study coordinator and the participant do not know whether they are in the intervention or usual care (placebo) group. This can be done with the help of a person independent of the trial who may make up courses of treatments in containers only identified by the trial number. Under these circumstances, this person would also hold the key to the allocation. Blinding reduces bias which may occur subconsciously, through the expectation that the intervention is more effective than usual care. This is relatively easy to do in drug trials whereby a new drug is being tested against the usual treatment, which may be no treatment.

In some studies it is possible to blind either the participant or researcher but not both. This is called single blind. With this level of blinding there is always a possibility that the blinded person discovers the treatment allocations. For example, participants may tell the researcher their allocation.

Example from the literature

A statistician not involved in the study carried out randomisation. Concealed envelopes were used to allocate the patients to either the occupational therapy or the control group and these envelopes were opened by an independent secretary. In this single blind randomised controlled trial, patients and care givers were aware of the treatment assigned. The assessors were blinded to group allocation. Patients and care givers were asked before each assessment not to inform the assessors about the intervention. To check the success or failure of the blinding after each measurement the assessors were asked if they had been told or knew for sure to which group each patient had been allocated. (Graff et al., 2006)

In the paper by Graff et al. (2006), the intervention was occupational therapy aimed at participants with dementia and their primary caregiver; the 'control' group received usual care. In this study, the researchers doing the outcome assessments were not aware of the group a given participant was randomised to, hence it was single blind. Participants and their caregivers could not be blinded to their allocation because they would be aware of whether they were receiving occupational therapy or not. Whether the blinding had been successful was reported as an outcome in this study.

A further example of the type of study that is difficult to blind is one where the intervention requires the participants to take part in an exercise programme. With this type of intervention the participants could not be blinded because they would know whether they are exercising or not, and from the participant information sheet they would know that the alternative would be no exercise related to the study. In this case it may be possible for the researchers who are assessing the participants' health to be blind to allocation if they are not involved in administering the intervention (and thus knowing which participants are allocated to which group). This also relies on participants not telling the researcher which group they have been randomised to.

In some studies the intervention is such that it is impossible to blind either the participants or the researchers. For example, in the United Kingdom Oscillation Study (UKOS) two types of ventilators were used to aid breathing in infants born extremely preterm (Johnson et al., 2002). The parents (a proxy for the infant in this example) and the health professionals knew which ventilator the infant had been randomised to. However, elements of the study were blinded. For example, chest x-rays were reviewed without the mode of ventilation being known.

Outcomes from randomised controlled trials can take a number of forms, which can be measured by the researcher or the participant. For example, in a randomised controlled trial where the intervention is exercise, the primary outcome may be weight change from baseline. Secondary outcomes may be more subjective such as quality of life at the end of the exercise programme.

Most randomised controlled trials are analysed using intention-to-treat. This means that participants are analysed in the group that they were randomised to regardless of whether they change to the other group during the course of the trial. This mimics what would take place in real life, with some people being offered a given treatment and within those some being compliant and others not. For example, in UKOS (Johnson et al., 2002) some infants changed from their randomised ventilator type to the other before the protocol permitted. However, statistical analysis was via intention to treat, that is, by randomised ventilator allocation. The alternative to this is per protocol which analyses participants by the treatment they actually received. This is more likely to show a difference in outcome than intention-to-treat.

The ethics of carrying out a randomised controlled trial must be carefully thought about. For example, it is unethical to randomise participants to a treatment or condition which it is known to be harmful; it would be unethical to randomise participants to smoking versus not smoking. Additionally, if there is an effective treatment for the condition of interest, then participants should not be left untreated. In this case the intervention would be the new treatment that is being tested which is compared to the usual effective treatment for the condition. During the course of randomised controlled trials, the ongoing results are monitored to ensure that one randomised treatment is not performing much better (or worse) than the other. If this is the case trials may be stopped to enable all participants to be able to receive the more beneficial treatment.

CLUSTER RANDOMISED TRIALS

Sometimes it is difficult to randomise individual participants to an intervention or treatment, such that it is easier and more appropriate to randomise whole groups to the intervention or usual treatment. This study design occurs when participants are being recruited to an intervention where participants can affect one another within a trial such as smoking cessation or weight loss. This may occur in GP practices, hospital wards or schools where, if participants were randomised individually they may influence the behaviour of one another. For example, the trial may be such that the same practice nurse administers the allocation or the intervention may be administered in groups. If participants were randomised individually, there is the possibility of the messages being polluted and participants receiving different allocations speaking to one another and incorporating parts of the other allocation into their lives. To avoid this everyone who participates in a study from a given GP practice receives the same allocation.

Additionally, those participants who come from the same source are more likely to be similar than those from elsewhere. For example, a participant who is registered at a given GP practice may be similar in terms of socioeconomic status and other demographic and/or social characteristics to any other person also registered at that GP practice compared with a participant registered at any other GP practice. This needs to be taken into consideration when calculating the sample size for the study. Furthermore, when the study is complete, non-independence of the data should be taken into account in statistical modelling. This can be done with methods such as generalised estimating equations or multilevel modelling, the detail of which is beyond the scope of this book, but further details on these types of analyses can be found in Donner and Klar (2000).

Example from the literature

> **Objective:** To evaluate a training programme intended to improve the management of obesity, delivered to general practice teams.
> **Design:** Cluster randomised trial.
> **Setting:** Northern and Yorkshire region of England.
> **Participants:** 44 general practices invited consecutively attending obese adults to participate; 843 patients attended for collection of baseline data and were subsequently randomised.

Intervention: 4.5 hour training programme promoting an obesity management model.

Main outcome measures: Difference in weight between patients in intervention and control groups at 12 months (main outcome measure) and at 3 months and 18 months; change in practitioners' knowledge and behaviour in obesity management consultations.

Results: Twelve months after training the patients in the intervention group were 1 (95% confidence interval −1.9 to 3.9) kg heavier than controls (P = 0.5). Some evidence indicated that practitioners' knowledge had improved. Some aspects of the management model, including recording weight, target weight, and dietary targets, occurred more frequently in intervention practices after the training, but in absolute terms levels of implementation were low.

Conclusion: A training package promoting a brief, prescriptive approach to the treatment of obesity through lifestyle modification, intended to be incorporated into routine clinical practice, did not ultimately affect the weight of this motivated and at risk cohort of patients. (Moore et al., 2003: 1085)

The study by Moore et al. (2003) randomised GP practices so that those attending a given GP practice got the same intervention or usual care. The intervention was delivered to the health professionals at the intervention practices. The fact that all relevant health professionals from the participating practices took part meant that participants should have received the same advice whoever they consulted in the practice. However, the results of this cluster randomised trial showed that the primary outcome was not significant '…the patients in the intervention group were 1 (95% confidence interval −1.9 to 3.9) kg heavier than controls (P = 0.5)' indicating that this approach to weight loss did not appear to be successful.

CROSSOVER TRIALS

Crossover trials are often used when the study population has a chronic condition, the intensity of which is unlikely to change over the duration of the trial such that participants can act as their own controls. It is possible for crossover trials to be double blind; participants are randomised to receive either the intervention or usual care first. This treatment will last for a specific length of time laid down in the protocol. At the end of the first treatment it may be necessary for there to be a washout period if the treatment is a drug or other form of medication whereby neither treatment is taken so that there are no residual effects of the first allocation when the second treatment commences.

It is possible to do crossover trials on technologies. For example, Wood and Lutman (2004) undertook a single blind crossover trial of analogue versus digital hearing aids. The advantage of using the same participants as their own controls in this study was that they are able to compare their hearing and quality of life with the two hearing aids. In this trial the participants were unaware of what type of hearing aid they were using, although the researchers were aware of allocation. Participants wore the analogue and digital hearing aids for five weeks each. Overall it was found that digital hearing aids were preferred to analogue hearing aids.

EXERCISES

Read the extracts below from the research papers and answer the questions related to them.

> For each bladder cancer case, one control was selected. Controls were individually matched to cases by age (within 5 years) at diagnosis/interview, gender, race/ethnicity and hospital. Controls were selected from patients admitted to the same hospital around the same time as the cases for diseases/conditions unrelated to the exposures under study. We identified 1465 eligible controls and interviewed 1271 (88%) of them (1105 men, 166 women). (Samanic et al., 2008)

1   Why were cases matched to controls?
2   What are the potential problems with matching?
3   Why were controls selected from the same hospitals as the cases but with diseases unrelated to that of the cases?

> The study population included 30 065 participants who were referred, during a five year period (2002–6), to the Institute of Sports Medicine to obtain eligibility to take part in competitive sports. All participants were examined with first line investigations, as required under Italian law. Since 1982, people participating in all officially sanctioned sports must undergo medical screening that includes personal and family history, physical examination, and resting and exercise 12 lead electrocardiography (ECG). (Sofi et al., 2008)

4   What type of study was this?
5   With this study, what are the disadvantages of the study design?

> A random number sequence and sealed numbered envelopes were generated by a statistician at the Cancer Research UK Medical Statistics Group, Oxford. Nurses opened the envelopes in sequence following eligibility assessment and consent. Participants attending together, such as husbands and wives, were allocated to the same arm. In some cases the envelopes were opened slightly out of sequence, which was inadvertent and not due to dislike of the allocation. The trial statistician was informed and was unconcerned. Participants and nurses were necessarily not blind to allocation although research staff making follow-up telephone calls at 3, 6 and 12 months were. (Aveyard et al., 2007)

6   What type of study is this?
7   What terms in the extract indicate what the study design is?
8   What might have been the effect on the study of opening envelopes out of sequence due to a dislike of the allocation?
9   What were the advantages of participants attending together being allocated in the same arm of the study?
10 If you wanted to carry out a study to determine the impact of a number of lifestyle factors over time, how would you do it? Include as much detail as possible.

4
PROBABILITY

INTRODUCTION

Whilst it may not be obvious how probability fits with health statistics, the concept of probability underlies all statistical tests, so a basic understanding of simple probability is essential so that it can be linked with these concepts. This chapter will start with defining probability using simple examples, which will then be broadened to show that simple probabilities can be used within routine health data. These concepts will be extended to the situation where two probabilities are considered: mutually exclusive events and independent events. Finally, probability will be linked to health statistics. This will be in the form of p-values.

THE AIMS OF THIS CHAPTER ARE:

- To learn what probability is.
- To learn the basic rules of probability.
- To link probability with health statistics.

WHAT IS PROBABILITY?

Probability is the proportion of times a given event will occur in the long run. This is not necessarily the proportion of times the event will occur in the short term because of random variation in the occurrence of events. For example, if a fair coin (that is, one which is equally likely to give a head or tail when tossed) is tossed and the first result is a head, all subsequent tosses could also be either a head or a tail, regardless of what the previous outcome was. It might be that a number of subsequent consecutive coin tosses produce the same as the first toss, but with increasing coin tosses this will even out and the proportion of heads will be 0.5 and the proportion of tails will be 0.5. This equates to a probability of one half for heads and one half for tails. These can also be presented as fractions or percentages, so the probability of getting a head in the long run is 0.5 (1/2 or 50%) and the probability of getting a tail in the long run is 0.5 (1/2 or 50%).

This is illustrated using data gained during a lecture whereby students were asked to toss a coin and then report the result when prompted to do so, this was done by row of the lecture theatre for ease of counting. The results of this exercise are shown in Table 4.1. It shows that overall 73 coins were tossed (shown at the bottom of the cumulative total column). All of the coins tossed by those on the first row of the

TABLE 4.1   RESULTS OF A COIN TOSSING EXERCISE

Row	Heads	Tails	Row % heads	Row % tails	Cumulative heads	Cumulative total	Overall % heads
1	0	4	0	100	0	4	0
2	4	2	67	33	4	10	40
3	1	7	14	86	5	18	28
4	4	4	50	50	9	26	35
5	4	3	57	43	13	33	39
6	4	1	80	20	17	38	45
7	6	3	67	33	23	47	49
8	3	2	60	40	26	52	50
9	4	7	36	64	30	63	47
10	5	5	50	50	35	73	48

lecture theatre produced tails, with subsequent rows showing differing percentages of heads and tails (as shown in the row percentages of heads and tails). Overall 35 heads were tossed, giving 48% of the total being heads. With increased coin tosses this would stabilise to 50% of the total being heads.

Probabilities are normally expressed as proportions. In terms of proportions they can range from 0 to 1; an event with a probability of 0 is never going to happen and an event with a probability of 1 is guaranteed to happen. Equally, the sum of all probabilities of a given event adds to one; that is one event will occur. For example, if a standard die is rolled, possible values are 1, 2, 3, 4, 5, 6. Each one of these has equal probabilities of occurring, that is 1/6 (0.17 or 17%). The probability is 1/6 because there are six possible values, all with the same probability of occurring:

$$1/6+1/6+1/6+1/6+1/6+1/6 = 1.$$

Examples of events with a probability of 0 are

- Rolling a 0 on a standard die – this is impossible because standard dice only have possible values of 1, 2, 3, 4, 5, 6.
- A human running a mile in 10 seconds – at present the male world record for a mile is 3:43.13 (IAAF, 2008), which is unlikely to reduce to 10 seconds considering human achievement to date and physiology to allow for potential improvement.

Examples of events with a probability of 1 are

- Rolling a 1, 2, 3, 4, 5 or 6 on a standard die – these are the standard numbers on a die, one of these will show when a standard die is rolled.
- Every human will die – no human lives forever, so the lifetime probability of death is 1.

A health related example

Using a more health related example, the probability of giving birth to a live male in the UK (disregarding other possible external factors) can be estimated from previous data collected by the Office for National Statistics (ONS, 2007b). In 2006, there were 669601 live births, of those 342429 were males. Therefore the estimated probability of giving birth to a live male is 342429/669601. This probability is hard to visualise as a fraction, so decimalising it gives a probability of 0.511 when expressed as a proportion or expressed as a percentage this is 51.1%; so excluding external factors, the estimated probability of giving birth to a live male in the UK is slightly higher than giving birth to a live female. The proportion of live births that were female can be calculated by subtraction as it is known that a live birth must be male or female and that the total proportion must be one. Therefore the proportion of female live births in 2006 was 1–0.511 = 0.489.

WHAT IF TWO EVENTS OCCUR?

Independent events

If one coin is tossed, and then tossed again, the result of the second coin toss is not influenced by that of the first, implying that the occurrence of the first event gives no information about the outcome of the second event. That means if, on the first coin toss the result is heads, the result of the second toss could be heads or tails. So the possible outcomes of tossing a coin twice are:

Heads – Heads   Heads – Tails   Tails – Heads   Tails – Tails

Each of these combinations are equally likely, so the probability of any of these combinations of two coin tosses occurring is one quarter (1/4, 0.25 or 25%). These are examples of independent events. The probability associated with tossing a head followed by a tail is:

Probability of tossing a head × probability of tossing a tail
1/2   ×   1/2
= 1/4

Note: when multiplying fractions, the numerators and denominators are each multiplied together. In the coin tossing example the two numerators are multiplied (1×1) and the two denominators are multiplied (2×2) to give $1/4$.

So to gain the probability of two independent events occurring, the individual probabilities should be multiplied by one another.

Another example

This principle can be extended to include a fair die and a fair coin. What is the probability of tossing a head on the coin and a 6 on the die? The probability of tossing a head is $1/2$ and the probability of throwing a 6 on the die is $1/6$. Therefore the probability is:

Probability of tossing a head $\times$ probability of throwing a 6
$1/2$ $\times$ $1/6$
$= 1/12$

MUTUALLY EXCLUSIVE EVENTS

Mutually exclusive means that if one event occurs, the other event cannot occur. This means that the probability being calculated is the probability that one event or the other occurs. The probability of a mutually exclusive event occurring is the sum of the individual probabilities. In the case where there are only two possible events and one of them must happen the probability is one; one event or the other will occur. For example, if a fair coin was tossed, the probability of getting a head or tail would be the sum of their individual probabilities, that is:

Probability of tossing a head $+$ probability of tossing a tail
$1/2$ $+$ $1/2$
$= 1$

Another example

If a fair die was thrown, the probability of getting each number $(1, 2, 3, 4, 5, \text{or } 6)$ is $1/6$. Therefore the probability of getting a five or six is:

Probability of getting a $+$ probability of getting a
5 on a fair die   6 on a fair die
$1/6$ $+$ $1/6$
$= 2/6 = 1/3$

HOW DOES THIS RELATE TO HEALTH STATISTICS?

Probability helps us consider the evidence available from the sample to make inferences about the population from which the sample is drawn. We do this by carrying out significance tests (explained in following chapters) and the measure of the strength of evidence is the p-value. A p-value is a probability. However, it is not the probability that the null hypothesis is not true (see Chapter 8 for an explanation of the null hypothesis), nor is it the probability that there is no difference between the groups being tested. It is actually the probability of obtaining a test statistic as extreme as that observed if there was no underlying difference or association in the population (that is, if the null hypothesis was true). As a p-value is a probability it takes values between 0 and 1. Most interest is derived (especially from non-statisticians) from p-values closer to 0 than 1. This is because those p-values less than 0.05 are termed 'statistically significant'. As a rule of thumb the following demarcations in p-values are used (Bland, 2000):

> Less than 0.01 – strong evidence of a difference or association.
> 0.01 to 0.05 – evidence of a difference or association.
> Less than 0.05 – a significant relationship has been shown.
> Greater than 0.1 – little or weak evidence of a difference or association.

As will be seen in later chapters of this book SPSS reports highly significant results as 0.000. In theory this is possible, but the exact p-value associated with that result is unlikely to be 0.000, so this should be reported as <0.001, since it is known that the result in question is <0.001, but without looking up the test statistic in a book of statistical tables the exact p-value is not known. However, when a result is highly significant like this, there is no real need to find out what the exact p-value is since for presentation purposes three decimal places are sufficient.

More details regarding test statistics and p-values will be given in later chapters of this book using SPSS examples.

SUMMARY

- The concept of probability is most commonly used in relation to statistics via p-values. However, it is useful to know some properties of probability, specifically the concepts of independent and mutually exclusive events.

EXERCISES

1 In 2005, 243324 males died (all cause, all ages) (ONS, 2007c). Of these 88292 died of diseases of the circulatory system (ICD10 I00 to I99). Of those who died what was the estimated proportion of males dying of a circulatory disorder in 2005?

2 In 2005, there were 841800 conceptions in the UK (ONS, 2007d): 185500 were to women aged 20 to 24 years and 211300 were to women aged 25 to 29 years. What was the estimated probability that a conception was to a woman in her twenties in 2005? (Note: data were reported to the nearest thousand by ONS).

3 Why might the probability calculated in Question 2 be incorrect?

4 Assuming no external influences and the proportion of males born does not change over time, use the proportion given earlier in this chapter to calculate the probability of a woman who has two live births having a male followed by a female.

5
SUMMARY STATISTICS FOR CONTINUOUS DATA

INTRODUCTION

Once the data are entered into SPSS it is good practice to plot continuous data; data that are either continuous or discrete and then obtain some descriptive statistics. These may reveal data that have not been entered correctly, and therefore need checking before further analysis can be carried out. For example, those who appeared over 100 years old may warrant further checking with the data collection sheet or the original source as there are few people in the population that old. Individual variables can be plotted using histograms. Histograms will also reveal the distribution of variables; useful for descriptive purposes and to determine which statistical tests are appropriate. Statistical tests are explained further in later chapters.

If data are entered correctly, summary statistics reveal the characteristics of the study participants. Regardless of the research question, descriptive statistics will undoubtedly be the initial results presented in a paper, report or thesis because the characteristics of the study population should be reported before more complex statistics are embarked upon and ultimately presented.

This chapter will utilise three datasets. The first is a student study of obesity (n=82), looking at factors that may contribute to obesity as well as participants' height and weight so that body mass index (BMI) could be computed. The second dataset is a study of knowledge of risk factors for type II diabetes in hotel workers (n=66); this study also collected data on height and weight so that BMI could be calculated. The final dataset to be used is the United Kingdom Oscillation Study (UKOS) (n=797); a randomised controlled trial of ventilation types for children born extremely preterm (Johnson et al., 2002).

THE AIMS OF THIS CHAPTER ARE:

- To look at the characteristics of single variables graphically to define the distribution of the variable.

- To summarise the data in terms of central tendency and spread.
- To learn how to obtain this information using SPSS.

PRELIMINARIES TO THIS CHAPTER

Before any graphs are invoked in SPSS, it is important that the type of data (that is, nominal, ordinal or scale) is declared correctly in Variable View. This is explained in Chapter 1.

HISTOGRAMS

Histograms display frequency distributions of continuous variables. The x-axis (horizontal) shows the continuous data whilst the y-axis (vertical) shows the frequency or percentage of the data. In SPSS the bars are called bins. The default number of bins and width of interval are determined by formula, but the number of bins can be altered by the user.

The data for this example are from a questionnaire on obesity. One of the questions asked the participants their height in either feet and inches or centimetres. The first example will use data from those who reported their height in centimetres.

To construct a histogram in SPSS, click on Graphs → Chart Builder... to get a dialog box like the one shown in Figure 5.1.

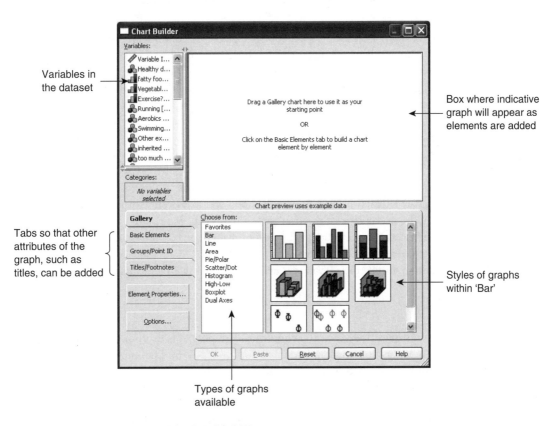

FIGURE 5.1   CHART BUILDER DIALOG BOX

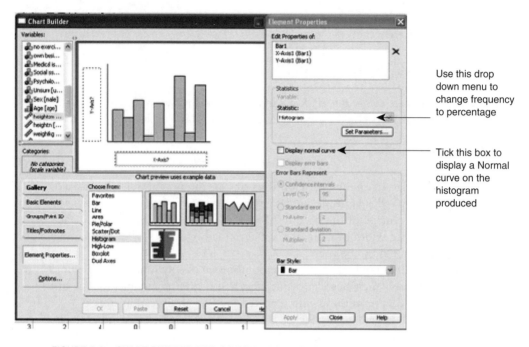

Use this drop down menu to change frequency to percentage

Tick this box to display a Normal curve on the histogram produced

FIGURE 5.2   CHART BUILDER DIALOG BOX WITH HISTOGRAM SELECTED

From the list of available graph types (under Choose from:), click on Histogram. The styles of histogram available will appear in the box next to the list of graph types. From the available styles, choose the one that appears in the top left corner of the style gallery (Simple Histogram) by dragging it to the chart preview box (the large white box above the style gallery). The Chart Builder dialog box then changes to look like Figure 5.2. To place the chosen variable on the x-axis, drag it from the Variables: box to the X–Axis? box. The Y–Axis box will change to Histogram. At this point, it is possible to click on OK to see the graph produced. Alternately, titles can be added using the appropriate tab on the left hand side of the dialog box. A Normal curve can be added by ticking the appropriate box (indicated in Figure 5.2) in the Element Properties dialog box (which opens next to the Chart Builder dialog box when a graph type has been selected). If instead of the frequency, the percentage of the data is required on the y-axis, this can be given by changing the Statistic: in the Element Properties dialog box to Histogram Percent then clicking Apply. Once the options have been selected, click OK on the Chart Builder dialog box. A histogram like the one illustrated in Figure 5.3 will be produced.

Interpretation

The histogram shows (in text to the right of the graphic, this is produced by default) the mean height was 163cm (standard deviation (SD) 37cm). The mean and standard deviation will be described further later in this chapter. There were a small number of very short people and one very tall person (bearing in mind it is known that the participants were human adults) whose height may require further investigation by checking the original questionnaires to discover whether there has been data entry error or the participant has answered the question incorrectly.

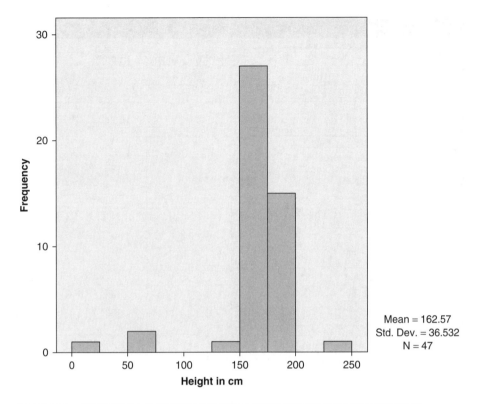

FIGURE 5.3   HISTOGRAM OF HEIGHT FOR THOSE WHO REPORTED THEIR HEIGHT IN CENTIMETRES

After further investigation it was found that the very small values were likely to be errors on the part of the participants. It is believed that these apparently short participants had filled in their feet and/or inches measurements in the space where height in centimetres was expected, but it was impossible to know this definitively. The very tall person was considered to be out of range, so was also excluded.

Editing graphs

It is possible to edit graphs. To do this, double click the histogram in the SPSS Viewer to invoke the Graph Editor, as in Figure 5.4.

When in the Graph Editor, double click on the part of the graph that requires changes. Both axes should be labelled for presentation (in Figure 5.4, the x-axis label should be better presented), these can be edited by double clicking on the label already there, then typing a replacement label. It is also possible to edit the colour of bars in histograms and bar charts and edit axis scales (the minimum, maximum and interval between markers on the y-axis of a histogram). It should be noted that the scales should be labelled appropriately, and that there is no need for a large number of decimal places to be displayed on graphics. In Figure 5.3, there is no need for any decimal places on either axis as human height is never measured more accurately

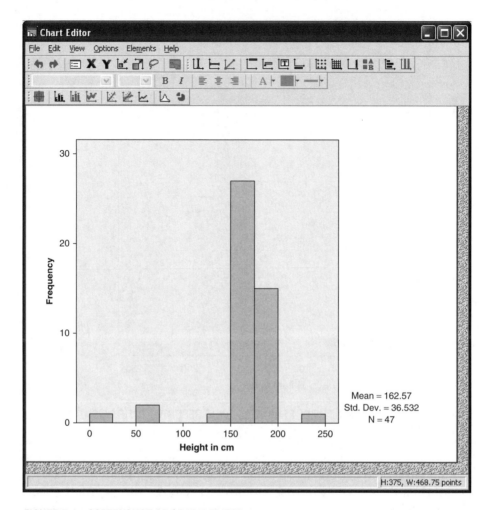

FIGURE 5.4   SCREENSHOT OF GRAPH EDITOR

than to the nearest centimetre and frequency can only be a whole number. Further conventions on presenting data are given by Freeman et al. (2008). The number of decimal places for the summary statistics placed next to the histogram cannot be changed, however, the summary statistics can be removed completely and the information conveyed with fewer decimal places in the text. When the graph has been edited, go to File → Close in the Graph Editor to return to SPSS Viewer. Figure 5.5 shows an edited graph.

A word of caution regarding out of range data

Data should not be deleted from a dataset unless there is good reason to do so. This means that everything possible should be done to check the data with the original

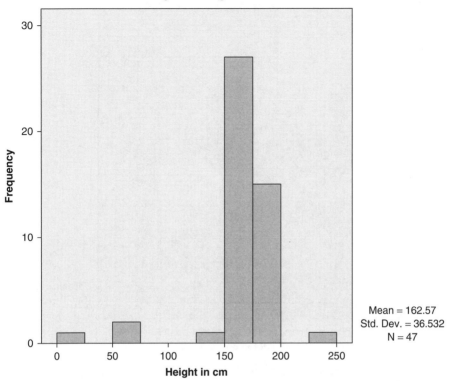

FIGURE 5.5   EDITED HISTOGRAM OF HEIGHT FOR THOSE WHO REPORTED THEIR HEIGHT IN CENTIMETRES

questionnaires, data extraction sheets or other sources. If a solution cannot be found, then it is permissible to delete individual values, although a record should be made of changes to the dataset so there is an audit trail of changes.

In Figures 5.3 and 5.5, it is clear there are some out of range heights, three below 100cm tall and one above 200cm tall. Figure 5.6 shows the same data with the extreme outliers removed. It can be seen that most people were between 160cm and 180cm whilst there were no participants more than 200cm tall or less than 100cm. The mean was 169cm (SD 13cm). Compared with the dataset with impossible values the mean height has increased by 6cm; however, a greater change has occurred to the standard deviation, which has decreased from 37cm in the dataset that included the out of range values to 13cm in the dataset without the out of range observations. The smaller standard deviation in the dataset with all values in range indicates that there is less variation in the data than there was in the variable as it was presented in Figures 5.3 and 5.5. There will be more about means and standard deviations later in this chapter. These results are more consistent with what is known about human height. When analysing your own data, it is likely you will know the range of values expected, so will know which values are highly unlikely to be true values.

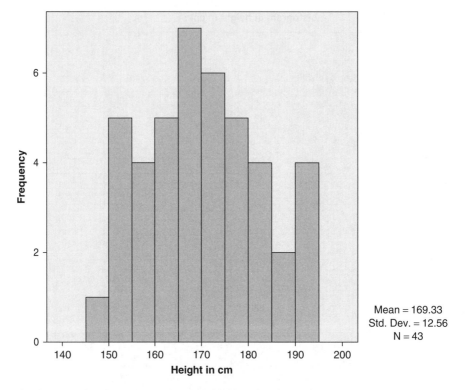

FIGURE 5.6   HISTOGRAM OF HEIGHT FOR THOSE WHO REPORTED THEIR HEIGHT IN CENTIMETRES WITHOUT THE OUT OF RANGE VALUES

HISTOGRAMS TO SHOW DISTRIBUTIONS

Histograms can also be used to show the distribution of variables visually. Looking at body mass index (BMI) from the obesity dataset, utilising data from all participants, gives the histogram shown in Figure 5.7. The mean BMI was 26kg/m² (SD 5kg/m²). This variable is positively skew (also known as right skew). This is characterised by a large number of lower value observations (shown by many participants with a lower BMI in this example) and few higher value observations (shown by the presence of fewer participants with a BMI over 35kg/m² in this example). This shape of distribution often occurs in depression scales (where 0 indicates no depression and a high score indicates severe depression) in a population sample of participants, whereby most people will not have depression, so will score close to zero, and a small number of people having severe depression and scoring very highly.

If there are a large number of higher value observations and few smaller observations, as in Figure 5.8, then the data are negatively skew (left skew). This shows gestational age in days of infants who were part of UKOS. It shows there were fewer infants born at lower gestational ages than higher gestational ages. The mean of this variable is 185 days (SD 10 days).

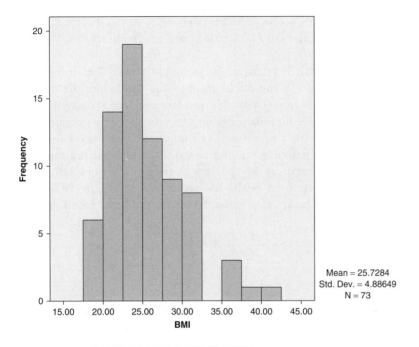

FIGURE 5.7   HISTOGRAM OF BODY MASS INDEX

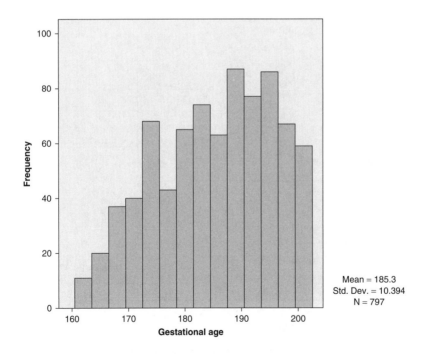

FIGURE 5.8   HISTOGRAM OF GESTATIONAL AGE IN THE UNITED KINGDOM OSCILLATION STUDY DATASET

The easiest way to remember the name for the direction of skew is that the direction of skew is the same side as the tail (where there are fewer observations) of the distribution.

The other distribution that is occasionally seen is bimodal. This distribution is characterised by two peaks in the distribution of the data when the data are plotted on a histogram. Sometimes, with this distribution there is an underlying reason for this occurrence. A bimodal distribution may appear to occur when the dataset is fairly small with a relatively large number of observations either side of the centre of the distribution giving two peaks when plotted on a histogram. Under these circumstances the apparent distribution may be influenced by the number of bins (bars) used in the histogram. A bimodal distribution is shown in Figure 5.9 using body mass index data from the hotel based diabetes awareness study.

Interpretation

Figure 5.9 shows that the mean body mass index (BMI) was 24.5kg/m^2 (SD 4.7kg/m^2). It shows that there are a large number of people with a BMI just over 20kg/m^2 and

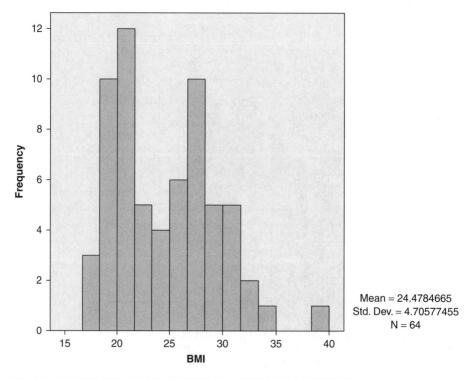

FIGURE 5.9   BODY MASS INDEX SHOWING A BIMODAL DISTRIBUTION

another peak between 25kg/m² and 30kg/m². It is likely this pattern is seen because of the relatively small sample size (n=64) as the apex of the peaks represent 12 and 10 participants respectively.

The distribution that is the most useful in statistical analysis is the Normal distribution. This is because the distribution forms part of the assumptions of many tests that will be described later in this book. This distribution is characterised by a small number of extremely low and high value observations, as shown in Figure 5.10 with a small number of observations less than −2 and greater than +2. Most observations are around the middle of the data range as shown by the large frequency around 0 (the mean in this example) in the simulated data shown in Figure 5.10 (SPSS Inc., 2007). Many human measurements such as height (if restricted to adults) and lung function follow the Normal distribution.

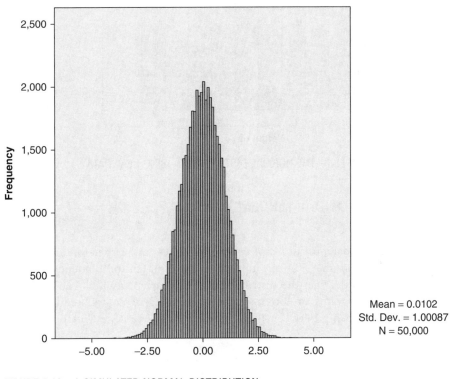

FIGURE 5.10   A SIMULATED NORMAL DISTRIBUTION

An example of real data with a Normal distribution is shown in Figure 5.11. It is all the height data (those reported in centimetres and feet and inches, after conversion to metres) from the obesity dataset. As these data are real, the distribution is not perfectly Normal, but can be considered to be so for analysis purposes.

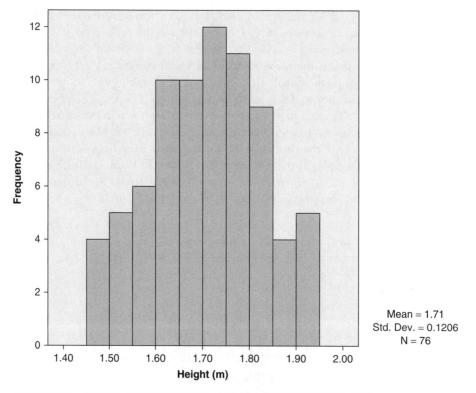

Mean = 1.71
Std. Dev. = 0.1206
N = 76

FIGURE 5.11   EXAMPLE OF THE NORMAL DISTRIBUTION USING REAL DATA

QUANTIFYING CENTRAL TENDENCY AND DISPERSION

With continuous data, measures of central tendency and dispersion are used to summarise each variable. The appropriate measure of central tendency for presentation is dependent on the distribution of the variable, which can be established using histograms or looking at the measures of central tendency and seeing the relationship between them. These will be explained further later in this chapter.

Central tendency

Mean

This is usually what people mean when they refer to the average. It is the sum of the observations within a variable divided by the total number of observations. Consider the following BMI data derived from the student obesity questionnaire (values have been rounded to the nearest integer):

20	31	25	22	24	25	32	28	31

There are nine observations shown; the sum of these is 238. Therefore the mean BMI is $26.4 kg/m^2$. This calculated by $(20+31+25+22+24+25+32+28+31)/9 = (238/9)$.

Median

This is the middle value when the observations in the dataset are put into order of magnitude. Taking the BMI data that were used to illustrate the mean:

20	31	25	22	24	25	32	28	31

These can be rearranged in order of magnitude giving:

20	22	24	25	<u>25</u>	28	31	31	32

As there are nine observations, the median will be the fifth observation from either end of the data series (underlined). Therefore, in this dataset, the median BMI is $25 kg/m^2$. This means that half the data in the dataset are below $25 kg/m^2$ and half the data are above $25 kg/m^2$. In this example there is another participant with a BMI of $25 kg/m^2$, this is shown below the median because the values are placed in ascending order.

The method of determining the median is slightly different if there is an even number of observations. In this case, the mean of the two middle observations is taken as the median. For example, if the BMI of one more person was calculated ($27 kg/m^2$), the dataset would consist of the following values:

20	31	25	22	24	25	32	28	31	27

If these are reordered by magnitude, the following ordering is obtained:

20	22	24	25	<u>25</u>	<u>27</u>	28	31	31	32

The middle two values in this dataset are 25 and 27 (underlined). The mean of these values is $(25+27)/2 = 26$. Therefore the median BMI of this dataset is $26 kg/m^2$. The mean of this dataset is $26.5 kg/m^2$ (265/10).

The relationship between the mean and median

When the data are Normally distributed, the mean and median are equal, and are located at the apex of a histogram of such a distribution. In Figure 5.10, the mean and median are zero. When the data are positively skew (right skew) as in Figure 5.7, the median will be less than the mean. In this example, the mean is $25.7 kg/m^2$ and the median is 24.8kg/m^2. The majority of the data are at the lower end of the range. As the median corresponds to the middle observation, this will be closer to the lower end of the range than the upper end. However, the mean will be higher because it will be influenced by the small number of higher valued observations. Conversely, if the data are negatively skew (left skew) as in Figure 5.8, the median will be higher than the mean because the majority of the data are higher valued observations and the mean will be influenced by the small number of lower valued observations. This is shown with the gestational age example, with the mean being 185 days and the median being 186 days.

Measuring dispersion

Range

The simplest way to measure dispersion is to give the range of the data; that is the difference between the largest and smallest observations. In the dataset of nine BMI observations used to illustrate the mean and median the range would be 32–20 = 12. SPSS would report the range for this dataset as 12. However, this does not tell us anything about the smallest and largest values as there are many ways which a range of 12 could be achieved. Therefore if the range is being reported it is more usual to give (minimum, maximum). In this dataset this would be (20, 32). The minimum and maximum can be obtained from SPSS. This will be shown later in this chapter.

<u>20</u>   22   24   25   25   28   31   31   <u>32</u>

The range can be useful but it depends only on the extreme values. These are likely to be further apart with larger sample sizes.

Interquartile range

To eliminate the dependence on the extreme values, the interquartile range is used as an alternative to the range. This is the difference between the first (lower quartile, (LQ)) and third (upper quartile, (UQ)) quartiles. The first quartile is the observation where 25% of the data are smaller than it (and 75% of observations are larger than it). The third quartile is the observation where 75% of the data are smaller than it. The interquartile range gives the range of values that are encompassed in the middle 50% of the dataset. The second quartile is the observation where 50% of the data are smaller than it. This is another name for the median. The interquartile range also requires the data to be ordered from smallest to largest if it is being calculated by hand (although in practice it is more likely a computer will do the computation, in which case the ordering does not matter). In the dataset of nine BMI measurements used earlier in this chapter, the lower quartile is 24, so that 25% of the data is below it. The upper quartile is 31; the point at which 25% of data are above it. The data are repeated with the upper and lower quartiles underlined.

		LQ		Median		UQ		
20	22	24	25	25	28	31	31	32

25% of
observations   25% of
observations

Sometimes the interquartile range is expressed as the upper quartile minus the lower quartile (UQ–LQ). In this example this would be 31–24=7. As with the range, a more informative way of expressing the interquartile range is (LQ, UQ). This gives (24, 31) for this example. This method of presentation is more informative than the subtraction method of presentation.

This principle can be extended to centiles (also called percentiles), whereby the dataset is divided into 100 equal parts. The principle is the same as for quartiles, with the lower quartile representing the 25th centile and the median representing the 50th centile. The 1st centile is the point below which 1% of the population lies. Other centiles can also be calculated or estimated using a cumulative percentage graph.

CUMULATIVE FREQUENCIES AND PERCENTAGES

Cumulative frequencies and percentages can be used with discrete or continuous data. Cumulative frequency is the number of observations within a variable that have values up to and including a given value, therefore data should be ordered in magnitude. This is illustrated in Figure 5.12 using apgar score one minute after birth from the United Kingdom Oscillation Study (n=782) (Johnson et al., 2002). This is a measure of well-being in infants

Apgar Score at one minute after birth

		Frequency	Percent	Valid Percent	Cumulative Percent
Valid	0	5	.6	.6	.6
	1	47	5.9	6.0	6.6
	2	55	6.9	7.0	13.7
	3	74	9.3	9.5	23.1
	4	98	12.3	12.5	35.7
	5	116	14.6	14.8	50.5
	6	117	14.7	15.0	65.5
	7	109	13.7	13.9	79.4
	8	91	11.4	11.6	91.0
	9	66	8.3	8.4	99.5
	10	4	.5	.5	100.0
	Total	782	98.1	100.0	
Missing	System	15	1.9		
Total		797	100.0		

FIGURE 5.12   FREQUENCY TABLE OF APGAR SCORE AT ONE MINUTE AFTER BIRTH

soon after birth. Figure 5.12 shows that the minimum is 0 and the maximum is 10, with the number with each individual score varying between 4 infants and 117 infants.

Cumulative frequency is calculated by taking the frequency of the lowest value (in Figure 5.12 this is 5 as there are five infants who had an apgar score of 0 – the lowest value). The frequency of the next highest observation is added to that to give the cumulative frequency for the first two values. Using Figure 5.12 this is 5+47, giving a cumulative frequency of 52 for an apgar score of 1. This procedure continues until the highest value within the variable has been reached. The cumulative frequency at this point will equal the total number of observations in the dataset (782 in Figure 5.12). Cumulative percentage follows the same principle using percentages rather than actual frequencies. The results of which are shown in Figure 5.12.

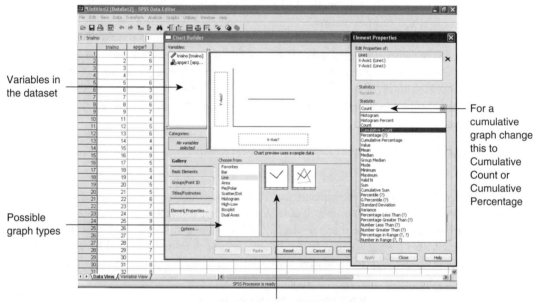

Variables in the dataset

For a cumulative graph change this to Cumulative Count or Cumulative Percentage

Possible graph types

Styles of graph available within the type chosen

FIGURE 5.13   CHART BUILDER DIALOG BOX WITH SIMPLE LINE GRAPH SELECTED

Once cumulative frequency or percentage values have been attained, they can be plotted on a cumulative frequency or percentage graph, with the variable values on the x axis (horizontal axis) and cumulative frequency or percentage on the y axis (vertical axis). These are achieved in SPSS by clicking on Graphs → Chart Builder... to get a dialog box as in Figure 5.1. From the Choose from: box highlight Line, then from the possible styles drag the one in the top left (Simple Line) to the large white box at the top of the dialog box, it will then change to look like Figure 5.13. From the list of variables in the dataset, move apgar1 to the x-Axis? box. To tell SPSS to give the cumulative frequency or cumulative percentage, from the Statistic: drop down box on the Element Properties dialog box select Cumulative Count or Cumulative Percentage as required. The interpolation type in Figure 5.14 was set at Step (the default is Straight), this can be changed in the Element Properties window. When all selections have been made, click OK. The resulting graphics can be seen in Figure 5.14.

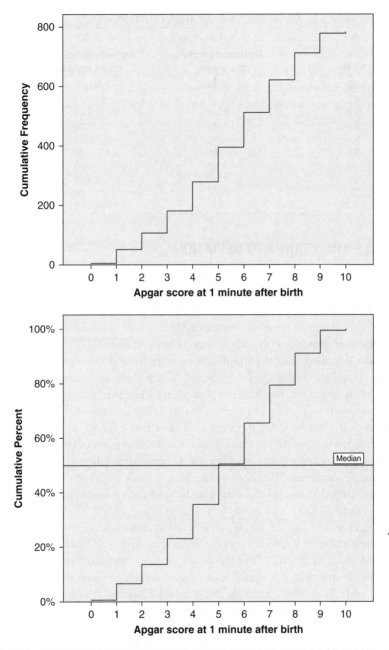

FIGURE 5.14   CUMULATIVE FREQUENCY AND CUMULATIVE PERCENTAGE OF APGAR SCORES ONE MINUTE AFTER BIRTH GRAPHS

Clearly these graphs (Figure 5.14) are the same shape as they are showing the same data, just expressing the cumulating in two ways. In the cumulative percentage graph, the median (the point where 50% of observations are smaller than the median and 50% of observations are larger than the median) has been marked with a horizontal line. The median apgar score is 5.

TABLE 5.1 EXAMPLE OF CALCULATION OF THE VARIANCE

A BMI	B Deviations from the mean	C Deviations from the mean squared
20	−6.44	41.53
22	−4.44	19.75
24	−2.44	5.98
25	−1.44	2.09
25	−1.44	2.09
28	1.56	2.42
31	4.56	20.75
31	4.56	20.75
32	5.56	30.86
Total	0.00	146.22

VARIANCE AND STANDARD DEVIATION

The variance is an estimate of variability of the data. It is calculated by subtracting the sample mean of the variable from each individual observation (For example, subtracting 26.44 from the nine observation BMI example used earlier in this chapter). These are called deviations from the mean (column B of Table 5.1). Those where the observation is smaller than the mean will be negative and those where the observation is larger than the mean will be positive. When these are summed they come to zero, which is of no use for further calculations. Therefore the deviations from the mean are squared and summed to give the sum of squares about the mean (Column C of Table 5.1). Finally, divide the sum of squares about the mean by the number of observations minus one (n−1), which is known as the degrees of freedom, to give the variance. In this example the number of degrees of freedom equals eight (9−1). Therefore the variance is 146.22/8 = 18.28.

For more information on the formulae behind the variance and degrees of freedom, see Bland (2000).

The variance is of limited use as a descriptive statistic because it is not in the same units as the variable of interest. It is in the units squared. In the BMI example the variance calculated is in $(kg/m^2)^2$. To give a statistic that is measured in the same units as the variable in question, the square root of the variance is taken to give the standard deviation (SD). In the BMI example the standard deviation is $\sqrt{18.28} = 4.28 kg/m^2$. If the SD is large in relation to the mean, it suggests the observations vary a lot, and if the SD is small in relation to the mean the observations vary little. Smaller SDs (relative to the mean) are usually seen with larger datasets.

The standard deviation has properties that relate to the Normal distribution. If the data are Normally distributed, 68% of the data will be within one standard deviation either side of the mean and 95% will be within two standard deviations of the mean, with 2.5% of the data at each extreme of the distribution. This is shown in the histogram of the Normal distribution in Figure 5.15. Therefore it is sometimes possible to infer whether a variable is Normally distributed from the mean and standard deviation. If the standard deviation is more than half of the size

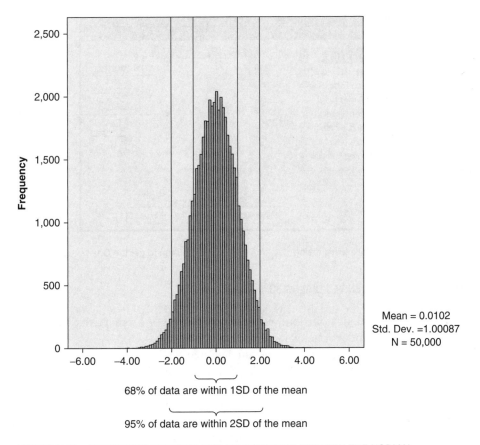

FIGURE 5.15   HISTOGRAM SHOWING THE RELATIONSHIP BETWEEN THE NORMAL DISTRIBUTION AND STANDARD DEVIATION

of the mean and negative values are impossible (for example height or weight, where it is impossible to be less than 0 tall or weigh less than 0 regardless of the units being used), then the distribution cannot be Normal. However, the reverse cannot be said to be true, that is, if the standard deviation is less than half the mean, it cannot be implied that the distribution is Normal. This is the case with the data presented thus far in this chapter.

FREQUENCY DISTRIBUTION

This is the set of all possible values for a given variable. Although the output can be long when used with continuous variables, it is worth doing as part of the data checking process, as this is an easy way of eliciting impossible values. In SPSS the Frequencies... command can also give summary statistics and histograms for continuous variables.

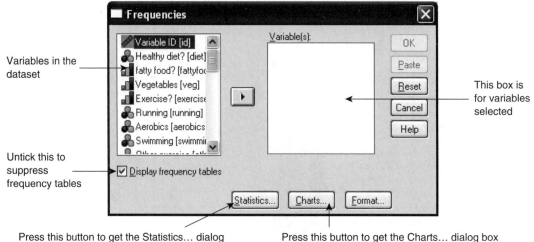

Variables in the dataset

Untick this to suppress frequency tables

This box is for variables selected

Press this button to get the Statistics... dialog box

Press this button to get the Charts... dialog box

FIGURE 5.16   FREQUENCIES DIALOG BOX

To obtain a frequency distribution, click on Analyze → Descriptive Statistics → Frequencies...to produce the dialog box shown in Figure 5.16.

Select the variable(s) that frequencies are required for. If more than one variable is required, hold the Ctrl button on the keyboard down and use the mouse to select the variables. Move the selected variable(s) to the box on the right called Variable(s): using the arrow button between the two boxes. It may not always be appropriate to display frequency tables for continuous variables, especially those that have a large number of data values because the tables are likely to be long and little useful information will be gained once the data cleaning process has been carried out. These can be suppressed by unticking the appropriate box (situated below the list of variables in the dataset) on the Frequencies dialog box (Figure 5.16).

Note: If a number of variables are selected at the same time, the same statistics and/or graphics will be produced for all variables, regardless of the appropriateness, therefore it is not good practice to use SPSS to summarise continuous and categorical variables at the same time. Categorical variables will be considered further in Chapter 6.

For continuous variables, it is useful to request some descriptive statistics by clicking the Statistics... button on the Frequencies dialog box. This will give the dialog box in Figure 5.17.

It is recommended that Quartiles, Mean, Median, Std. Deviation, Minimum and Maximum are selected by placing ticks next to the appropriate statistical function. When the selection has been made click Continue to return to the Frequencies dialog box (Figure 5.16).

A histogram to show the distribution of the variable may also be required. This can be requested by clicking on the Charts... button from within the Frequencies dialog box to give the Frequencies: Charts dialog box (Figure 5.18).

The default is not to produce any charts. To request a histogram, click on the Histograms: radio button. It is possible to add a Normal curve to the histogram with the same mean and standard deviation as the variable in question, by ticking the With

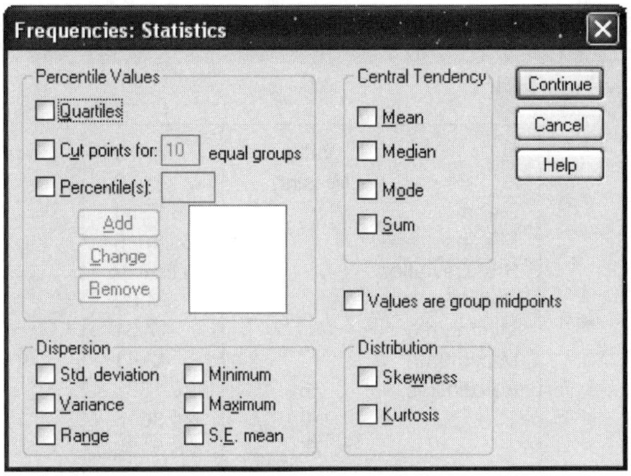

FIGURE 5.17   FREQUENCIES: STATISTICS DIALOG BOX

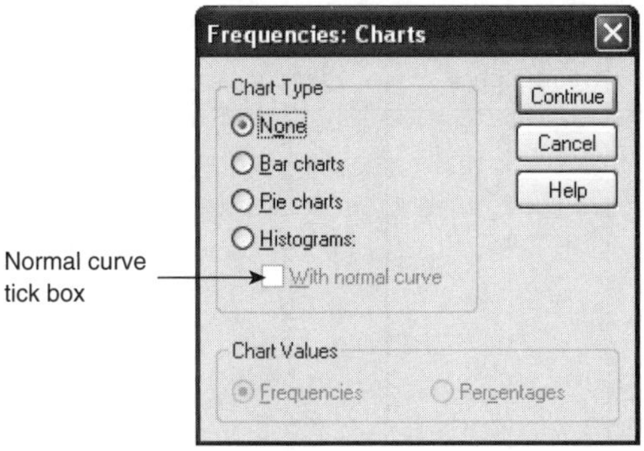

Normal curve
tick box

FIGURE 5.18   FREQUENCIES: CHARTS DIALOG BOX

normal curve box. Then click Continue to return to the Frequencies dialog box (Figure 5.16) then click OK.

Using the obesity data used previously in this chapter, and specifically the variable relating to BMI, the results from using the Frequencies… command are shown in Figure 5.19.

Interpretation

In this dataset, the mean body mass index (BMI) was 25.7kg/m^2 (SD 4.97kg/m^2). The minimum BMI was 17.6kg/m^2, and the maximum 42.4kg/m^2. The data are positively (right) skewed.

These data should be extracted from the SPSS output. SPSS output should not be copied and pasted directly into reports, dissertations or theses. Where there are a number of results to be conveyed (which may not all be explained in the text) the required statistics should be extracted and put into a table. Ways to do this clearly are given by Freeman et al. (2008).

Statistics

BMI

N	Valid	73
	Missing	9
Mean		25.7284
Median		24.8016
Std. Deviation		4.88649
Range		24.80
Minimum		17.61
Maximum		42.41
Percentiles	25	22.1838
	50	24.8016
	75	28.2132

BMI

		Frequency	Percent	Valid Percent	Cumulative Percent
Valid	17.61	1	1.2	1.4	1.4
	19.33	1	1.2	1.4	2.7
	19.39	1	1.2	1.4	4.1
	19.48	1	1.2	1.4	5.5
	19.59	1	1.2	1.4	6.8
	19.63	1	1.2	1.4	8.2
	20.28	1	1.2	1.4	9.6
	20.72	1	1.2	1.4	11.0
	20.78	2	2.4	2.7	13.7
	21.37	1	1.2	1.4	15.1
	21.75	1	1.2	1.4	16.4
	21.91	1	1.2	1.4	17.8
	21.97	1	1.2	1.4	19.2
	22.04	1	1.2	1.4	20.5
	22.09	1	1.2	1.4	21.9
	22.14	1	1.2	1.4	23.3
	22.15	1	1.2	1.4	24.7
	22.22	1	1.2	1.4	26.0
	22.49	1	1.2	1.4	27.4
	22.51	1	1.2	1.4	28.8
	22.58	1	1.2	1.4	30.1
	22.79	1	1.2	1.4	31.5
	22.83	1	1.2	1.4	32.9
	22.86	1	1.2	1.4	34.2
	23.01	1	1.2	1.4	35.6
	23.24	1	1.2	1.4	37.0
	23.30	1	1.2	1.4	38.4
	23.37	1	1.2	1.4	39.7
	23.46	1	1.2	1.4	41.1
	23.62	1	1.2	1.4	42.5

(Continued)

(Continued)

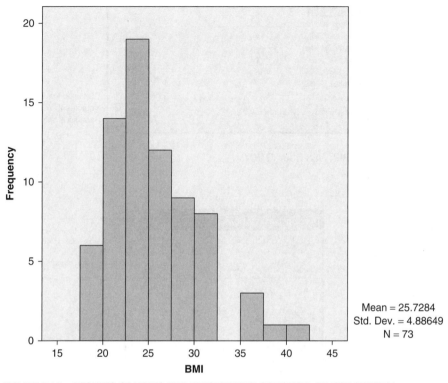

Mean = 25.7284
Std. Dev. = 4.88649
N = 73

FIGURE 5.19   RESULTS OF USING THE FREQUENCIES COMMAND ON THE OBESITY
DATA'S BODY MASS INDEX VARIABLE

DESCRIPTIVE STATISTICS

Sometimes the only statistics that are required are the descriptive statistics (that is, no frequency table). Although the frequency table can be suppressed in the Frequencies… command, Descriptives… can be used as an alternative under these circumstances (although as shown in Figure 5.21, possible statistics from this function are limited). To invoke the Descriptives dialog box shown in Figure 5.20, click on Analyze → Descriptive Statistics → Descriptives….

Transfer the variable(s) that descriptive statistics are required for into the large box. On clicking the Options… button, the Descriptives: Options dialog box shown in Figure 5.21 appears. The descriptive statistics ticked in Figure 5.21 are the default ones; others can be added by ticking the appropriate boxes.

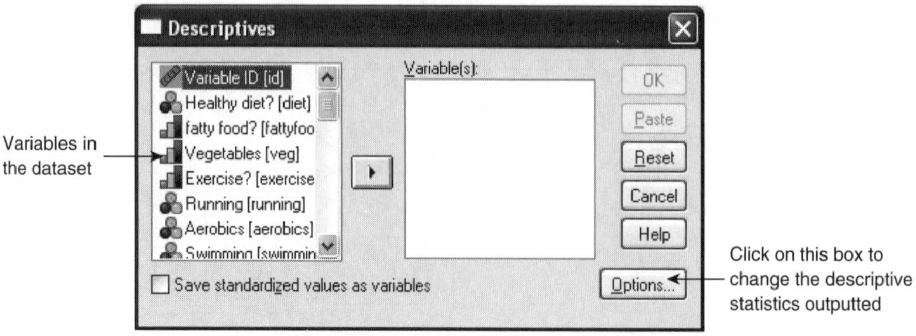

FIGURE 5.20 DESCRIPTIVES DIALOG BOX

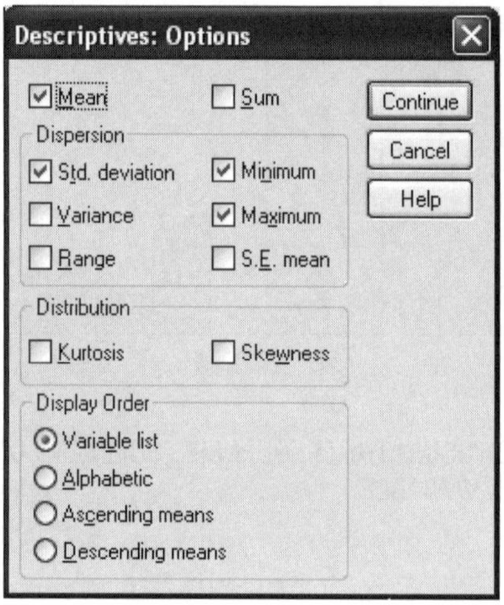

FIGURE 5.21 DESCRIPTIVES: OPTIONS DIALOG BOX

When the descriptive statistics required have been requested, click Continue to return to the Descriptives dialog box (Figure 5.20), then click OK. The results shown in Figure 5.22 have utilised the same dataset and variable (body mass index) as shown in Figure 5.19.

Descriptive Statistics

	N	Minimum	Maximum	Mean	Std. Deviation
BMI	73	17.61	42.41	25.7284	4.88649
Valid N (listwise)	73				

FIGURE 5.22 BODY MASS INDEX DESCRIPTIVE STATISTICS

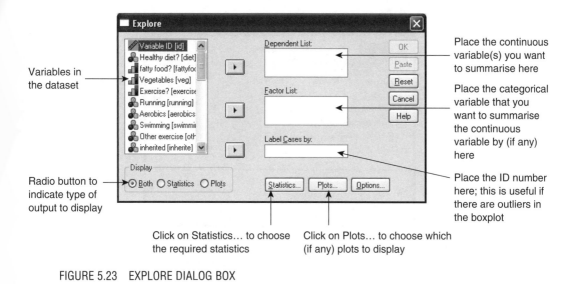

Variables in the dataset

Place the continuous variable(s) you want to summarise here

Place the categorical variable that you want to summarise the continuous variable by (if any) here

Radio button to indicate type of output to display

Place the ID number here; this is useful if there are outliers in the boxplot

Click on Statistics... to choose the required statistics

Click on Plots... to choose which (if any) plots to display

FIGURE 5.23   EXPLORE DIALOG BOX

EXPLORE

Explore can be used to give a variety of summary statistics and graphical representations. It can be used to give summary statistics for a continuous variable by a categorical variable, which may be useful for checking consistencies between two variables. For example, in a dataset containing gender and number of pregnancies, this should be missing (not applicable) for males. This could be checked using Explore to ensure there are no data present for males. To invoke Explore, click Analyze → Descriptive Statistics → Explore... to give the Explore dialog box in Figure 5.23.

The continuous variables to be summarised should be transferred to the Dependent List: box and the categorical variable which the data are to be summarised by should be transferred to the Factor List: box. The statistics required can be selected by clicking the Statistics... button to give the Explore: Statistics dialog

FIGURE 5.24   EXPLORE: STATISTICS DIALOG BOX

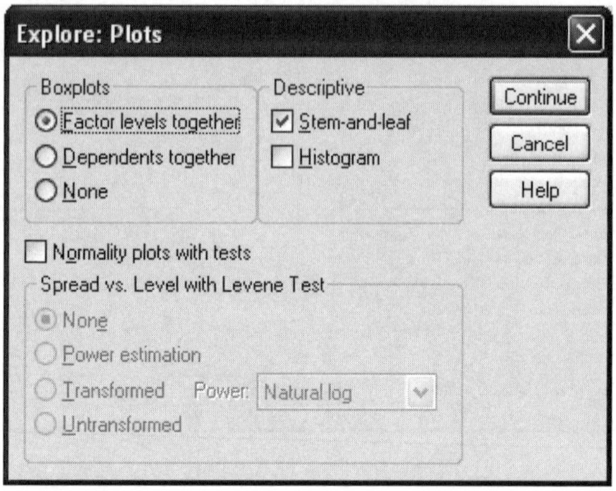

FIGURE 5.25   EXPLORE: PLOTS DIALOG BOX

box as shown in Figure 5.24. The default is Descriptives; it may also be useful to tick Percentiles. When statistics have been selected, click Continue to return to the Explore dialog box (Figure 5.23).

Likewise, if graphics are required, click the Plots… button to get the Explore: Plots dialog box shown in Figure 5.25. Boxplots and stem–and–leaf plots are the defaults; histograms can be added by ticking the appropriate box. Then click Continue to return to the Explore dialog box (Figure 5.23), and then click OK.

This example will continue to use the body mass index variable from the obesity dataset. This will be shown by sex to demonstrate how this function can be used to give descriptive statistics by a categorical variable. To do this, put BMI in the Dependent List: box, sex in the Factor List: box and ID number in the Label Cases by: box. The variable selected as Label Cases by: will be used in the boxplot to identify extreme data points.

Interpretation

In Figure 5.26a, it can be seen that there are 42 females and 31 males with data for both sex and BMI. Moving onto the descriptive statistics (Figure 5.26b), the mean BMI for females was 26.2kg/m² (SD 5.6kg/m²); whilst for males it was 25.1kg/m² (SD 3.6kg/m²). The minimum BMI for females was lower than for males (17.6kg/m² versus 19.4kg/m²) whilst the maximum BMI for females was higher than for males (42.4kg/m² versus 32.2kg/m²).

Figure 5.26c shows a stem–and–leaf plot, another way to display data to see its distribution, as it is essentially a low tech histogram rotated 90°. The stem has been indicated on the female plot with the smaller box. This consists of the first digit (the 'tens') of the BMI. In the smaller box there are two '2', the first one represents BMI from 20.00kg/m² to 24.99kg/m², and the second one represents BMI from

Case Processing Summary

		Cases					
		Valid		Missing		Total	
	Sex	N	Percent	N	Percent	N	Percent
BMI	Female	42	89.4%	5	10.6%	47	100.0%
	Male	31	91.2%	3	8.8%	34	100.0%

FIGURE 5.26A   CASE PROCESSING SUMMARY FOR BODY MASS INDEX BY SEX

Descriptives

	Sex			Statistic	Std. Error
BMI	Female	Mean		26.1890	.87117
		95% Confidence	Lower Bound	24.4296	
		Interval for Mean	Upper Bound		
				27.9484	
		5% Trimmed Mean		25.8103	
		Median		24.8893	
		Variance		31.875	
		Std. Deviation		5.64582	
		Minimum		17.61	
		Maximum		42.41	
		Range		24.80	
		Interquartile Range		7.00	
		Skewness		1.081	.365
		Kurtosis		.904	.717
	Male	Mean		25.1044	.64868
		95% Confidence	Lower Bound	23.7797	
		Interval for Mean	Upper Bound		
				26.4292	
		5% Trimmed Mean		25.0219	
		Median		24.4857	
		Variance		13.044	
		Std. Deviation		3.61170	
		Minimum		19.39	
		Maximum		32.24	
		Range		12.85	
		Interquartile Range		4.87	
		Skewness		.459	.421
		Kurtosis		−.590	.821

FIGURE 5.26B   DESCRIPTIVES FOR BODY MASS INDEX BY SEX

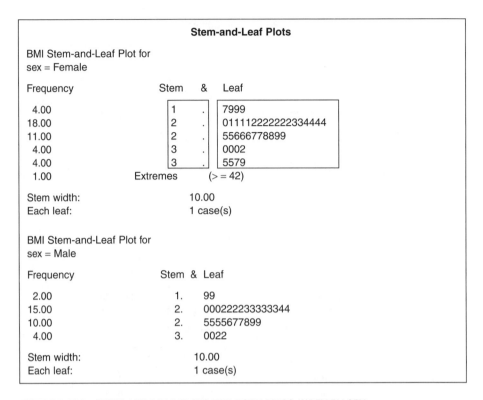

FIGURE 5.26C   STEM-AND-LEAF PLOTS FOR BODY MASS INDEX BY SEX

25.00kg/m^2 to 29.99kg/m^2. Those data in the larger box are representative of the 'units'. For example, after the '1' in the smaller box there is 7999 in the larger box, these represent four BMI scores of 17, 19, 19, 19. Note: underneath the final stem is indicated that there is one extreme BMI greater than 42kg/m^2. Similar interpretations can be drawn from the stem–and–leaf plot for males. Stem–and–leaf plots are not usually included in final reports, theses or dissertations. They are usually used to look for patterns in the data.

Figure 5.26d shows boxplots, another graphical representation of the data for males and females separately. The horizontal lines going through the boxes represent the medians, with the upper and lower boundaries of the boxes representing the upper and lower quartiles respectively. Therefore the length of the box equals the interquartile range. The lines coming out of the top and bottom of the boxes are known as the whiskers (these are sometimes called box and whisker plots). These extend for a maximum of 1.5 times the boxes' length, or to the minimum or maximum (whichever is shortest). Above the boxplot for females in Figure 5.26d is a circle with a number (the ID number). This is an outlier. Very extreme values are indicated with a star (there are none in Figure 5.26d).

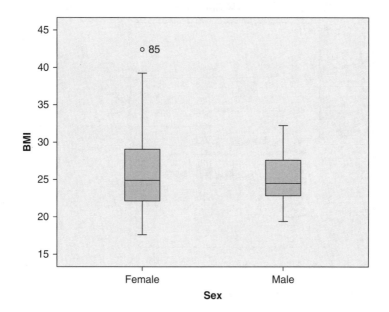

FIGURE 5.26D   BOXPLOTS FOR BODY MASS INDEX BY SEX

BOXPLOTS

Boxplots can also be created through the Chart Builder, so that only a boxplot (without the statistics) is produced. This will be illustrated with the same data as for Explore; namely BMI and sex. Firstly invoke the Chart Builder by clicking on Graphs → Chart Builder... to get the dialog box shown in Figure 5.1. From the list under Choose from: highlight Boxplot, then drag the Simple Boxplot icon (the one in the top left) to the large white box so that the Chart Builder looks like Figure 5.27. Into the Y-Axis? box drag the continuous variable (BMI) and drag the categorical variable (sex) into the X-Axis? box. To identify the outliers in a meaningful way, click on the Groups/Point ID tab, then tick Point ID Label so that the Point Label ID? Box appears in the large white box where the indicative boxplot is situated. Drag the participant identifier to this box. If the participant identifier is used as the identifying variable then it is easy to determine which participant has provided measurements that are different to the majority. If no identifying variable is declared then outliers are identified by the grey numbers on the left of Data View. These can change if data are sorted so an individual participant is not easily identified. Then click OK to give the same boxplots as shown in Figure 5.26d.

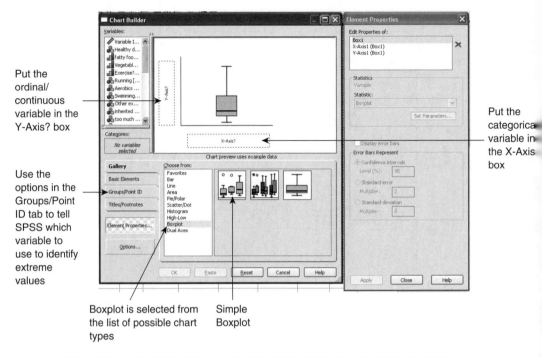

Put the ordinal/continuous variable in the Y-Axis? box

Put the categorical variable in the X-Axis box

Use the options in the Groups/Point ID tab to tell SPSS which variable to use to identify extreme values

Boxplot is selected from the list of possible chart types

Simple Boxplot

FIGURE 5.27   CHART BUILDER DIALOG BOX AFTER BOXPLOT HAS BEEN SELECTED

SUMMARY

- It is important to do summary statistics to discover the characteristics of the dataset. The type of summary statistics used will depend on the type of data to be summarised.
- Mean and median are commonly used measures of central tendency whilst standard deviation, range and interquartile range are used to indicate the spread of the data. Mean is usually accompanied by the standard deviation and median by the range or interquartile range.
- Frequencies can be computed by going to Analyze → Descriptive Statistics → Frequencies….
- Descriptive statistics for continuous variables can be invoked using Analyze → Descriptive Statistics → Descriptives….
- The Explore command can be used to give summary statistics for a continuous variable by a given categorical variable. This is given from Analyze → Descriptive Statistics → Explore….
- Boxplots and histograms can be drawn using: Graphs → Chart Builder… then selecting the appropriate options.

EXERCISES

1 In a study of infants treated for congenital diaphragmatic hernia in one hospital between 1996 and 2005, the mean birthweight was 3051g (SD 686g, n=44) and the mean number of days to surgery was 9.6 (SD 11.5, n=33) (Ng et al., 2008). What can be inferrred about the distributions of these data from these summary statistics?
2 Interpret the Stem-and-Leaf plot in Figure 5.26c for males.

6
SUMMARY STATISTICS FOR CATEGORICAL DATA

INTRODUCTION

Just as it is important to summarise continuous variables, it is also important to summarise categorical data; for example variables which show ethnicity, religion, disease status or smoking status. As with continuous data, entry errors can be found through looking at frequency tables. These will be revealed by an unexpected numerical code which does not correspond to any code assigned to that variable. Rogue values should be checked and the correct value inserted if possible. Sometimes errors are due to pressing the wrong key during data entry; or else they could be as a result of filling the wrong cell when there are missing data in adjacent cells (a reason for including a missing data code – meaning that all cells are then filled).

Categorical data are not usually presented graphically in assignments, dissertations, theses or papers because they take a large amount of space for the amount of information they are conveying. However, it may be necessary to present categorical data graphically for oral presentations or posters. To this end bar charts and pie charts are included in this chapter.

The data used in this chapter comes from a survey of younger (18 to 49 years) women's awareness of breast cancer risk factors and symptoms by ethnicity and age group. Ethnicity was collected in a large number of categories which were condensed to three – white, black or other – because there were little data from people of some ethnic groups.

THE AIMS OF THIS CHAPTER ARE:

- To understand how to obtain summary statistics for categorical variables using SPSS.
- To interpret summary statistics for categorical data.
- To graphically display categorical data.

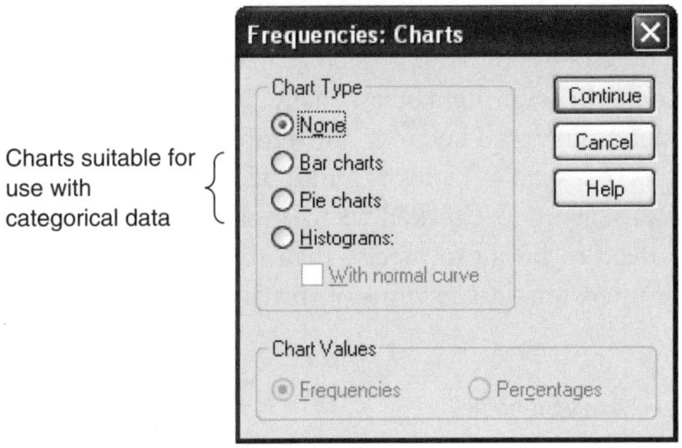

Charts suitable for use with categorical data

FIGURE 6.1   FREQUENCIES: CHARTS DIALOG BOX

FREQUENCIES

In SPSS frequencies are requested to get summary statistics for categorical data as for continuous data. However, it is not necessary to request histograms or statistics from categorical data because they would be meaningless. The frequency table is of key interest. This gives the frequency that a given category occurs in the dataset along with the percentage of the total that this represents. These can be gained by clicking on Analyze → Descriptive Statistics → Frequencies…. The dialog box is the same as for continuous data (Chapter 5, Figure 5.16).

The Charts… button gives a dialog box with options to produce bar and pie charts (Figure 6.1). These give an indication of the numbers and/or percentages in each category. However, they should not be used when there are a very small number of categories within a variable because such a graphic will not show anything meaningful. For example, a pie chart showing sex will not show anything meaningful, especially when the data come from a population sample so there is approximately 50% of participants in each category. When using Frequencies to obtain graphs, it is only possible to obtain one type of graph with each execution of the command; that is, only bar charts or pie charts can be produced at any one time. When a chart type has been selected (if any), click the Continue button to return to the Frequencies dialog box. More information can be found on bar and pie charts later in this chapter.

A diversion to percentages and proportions

This section serves as a reminder of and an extension to what was introduced in Chapter 4. Percentages are the key way of presenting categorical data. Percentages are calculated by dividing the number of participants with a given characteristic (the numerator) by the total number of participants with data present (the denominator) and multiplying by 100. The percentages of all possible categories in a dataset will add to 100%. If the result of the division is not multiplied by 100, then it is known as the proportion of respondents with a given characteristic. For example, in Figure 6.2, nine of 162 women checked their breasts daily. In this example 9 is the numerator and 162 is the denominator. Therefore the proportion of women checking their breasts daily was 9/162 = 0.06. If this is multiplied by 100 to give the percentage, it will show that 6% of women checked their breasts daily. When reporting percentages, there is no need to be more precise than the nearest whole percentage as has been done in the interpretation sections of this and later chapters.

Statistics
how often do you check your breast

N	Valid	162
	Missing	0

How often do you check your breasts?

		Frequency	Percent	Valid Percent	Cumulative Percent
Valid	daily	9	5.6	5.6	5.6
	at least once a week	26	16.0	16.0	21.6
	at least once a month	45	27.8	27.8	49.4
	at least once every 6 months	20	12.3	12.3	61.7
	not as often as every 6 months	31	19.1	19.1	80.9
	never	31	19.1	19.1	100.0
	Total	162	100.0	100.0	

How often do you check your breasts?

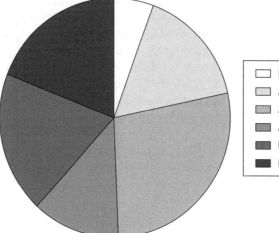
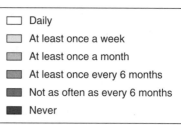

FIGURE 6.2   EXAMPLE OF FREQUENCY OUTPUT USING CATEGORICAL DATA – 'HOW OFTEN DO YOU CHECK YOUR BREASTS?'

Another diversion: missing data

In most datasets, some variables have missing data, which provides no information on the variable in question, so these participants should not be taken into account when doing any analyses. SPSS gives percentages that include and exclude missing data; it calls these Percent and Valid Percent respectively. Valid Percent should be presented. Of course, where there are no missing data, Percent and Valid Percent will be the same.

Missing data can come about in a number of ways. The most obvious way is through the information not being collected at the data collection stage of the study. This can be because the information was not filled in on the questionnaire, maybe the information requested was considered personal and the respondent did not want to divulge such information. For example, some people may not answer questions on such subjects as sexual behaviour despite assurances that the data they provide will be treated in the strictest of confidence. Alternately a large section of a questionnaire may have been omitted because the respondent did not turn the page to reveal further questions. It is possible to reduce this form of missing data by providing clear signposts as to the layout of the questionnaire and where the next questions are located or minimising the length of a questionnaire to keep it to one side of paper. Missing data can also occur when participants are being examined as part of a research study; for example, participants may find a given test painful to complete or they may opt out of blood testing meaning that all data that would have been generated as a result of analysing the blood will be missing.

Data can also appear to be missing in a datasheet because the question was not relevant to some respondents. The information elicited from these types of questions may only be relevant if participants fulfil some criteria such as having a particular medical condition, therefore those without the condition would not have the relevant knowledge or opinions to answer subsequent related questions. For example, the breast cancer awareness survey asked whether respondents knew anyone who had breast cancer, with a following question to elicit the relationship between the respondent and the person with breast cancer. Clearly, only those who knew someone with breast cancer could answer the subsequent question.

Finally, missing data is common in cohort (longitudinal) studies where participants drop out of the study, meaning that no data may be collected from some participants at some time points. Missing data usually increases with increasing time since the study began, which could be for a number of reasons, including not wanting to take part in the study any longer, death or moving away from the study area. Missing data in these circumstances can have consequences for the study population; those that drop out of such studies may have different characteristics than those who remain in the study.

Returning to frequencies

Statistics

know anyone who has breast cancer

N	Valid	161
	Missing	1

know anyone who has breast cancer

		Frequency	Percent	Valid Percent	Cumulative Percent
Valid	no	70	43.2	43.5	43.5
	yes	91	56.2	56.5	100.0
	Total	161	99.4	100.0	
Missing	System	1	.6		
Total		162	100.0		

FIGURE 6.3   EXAMPLE OF FREQUENCY OUTPUT USING CATEGORICAL DATA – 'DO YOU KNOW ANYONE WHO HAS/HAD BREAST CANCER?'

Interpretation

Figure 6.2 shows that 162 women responded to this question. It found that 45 women (28%) checked their breasts at least once a month, but less than once a week. Sixty-two women (38%) checked their breasts once a year or less. The pie chart represents the data in the table graphically. It can be seen that the largest segment (indicating the largest number (percentage) of women giving that response was for 'at least once a month' but less than once a week, whilst the smallest segment was for 'daily').

The variable 'How often do you check your breasts?' (Figure 6.2) did not have any missing data, so Percent and Valid Percent were the same. However, in Figure 6.3 there was one respondent who did not answer the question regarding whether they know anyone who has/had breast cancer, meaning that Percent and Valid Percent are different. Valid Percent should be used. In this example the difference in percentages between Percent and Valid Percent is very small; however, where there are a lot of missing data, or where the dataset is small and there are missing data, Percent and Valid Percent will differ considerably.

Interpretation

Fifty-seven percent of women (91/161) knew someone who has/had breast cancer.

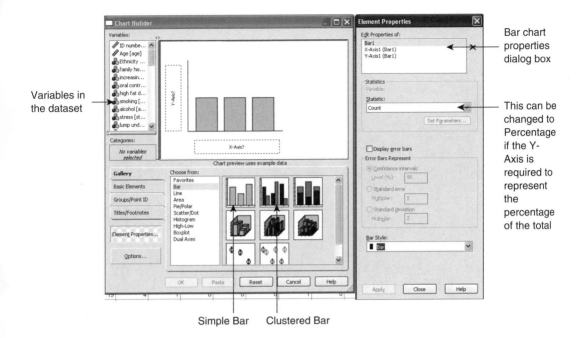

FIGURE 6.4   CHART BUILDER DIALOG BOX WITH BAR CHART SELECTED

BAR CHARTS

Bar charts graphically display variables containing nominal data, showing the percentage or frequencies (called Counts in SPSS graphics) of respondents who fall into each category. As explained earlier in this chapter, simple bar charts can be produced through the Frequencies command.

To generate bar charts without having to use Frequencies or to produce more complex bar charts, click on Graphs → Chart Builder…. From the Choose from: list highlight Bar then drag the Simple Bar diagram to the Chart Preview area, at which point the dialog box will look like Figure 6.4. Then drag the categorical variable of interest to the X-Axis? box. The box labelled Y-Axis? in Figure 6.4 will change to Count once an x-axis variable has been declared. This can be changed to percentage by changing the Statistic: in the Element Properties dialog box (Figure 6.4). When all submissions have been made to define the chart (including titles and labels as appropriate), click OK on the dialog box in Figure 6.4 to produce a bar chart like that in Figure 6.5. This example relates to 'How often do you check your breasts?'

Interpretation

The bar chart shows that more than 40 women in the study check their breasts at least once a month (but less than once a week), whilst fewer than 10 check their breasts daily. More than 30 women never check their breasts.

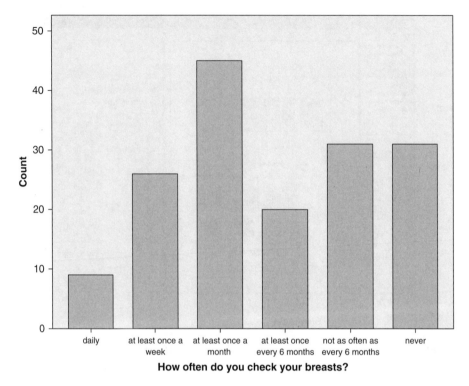

FIGURE 6.5   EXAMPLE OUTPUT FOR 'HOW OFTEN DO YOU CHECK YOUR BREASTS?'

It is worth noting that interpretation may be easier if data in bar charts are presented using percentages of the total. Percentages can be requested from the Element Properties dialog box (shown at the same time as the Chart Builder dialog box, Figure 6.4 indicates which element should be changed).

CLUSTERED BAR CHARTS

To construct a bar chart of a variable by another categorical variable, drag Clustered Bar to the large white box in the Chart Builder dialog box to define the type of bar chart (clustered bar type is pointed out in Figure 6.4). This will give the dialog box shown in Figure 6.6. As in the previous example, drag the main variable of interest (in this case How often do you check your breast?) to the X-Axis? box. The variable that this is going to be clustered by should be dragged to the Cluster: set color box. This example will use ethnic group in three categories. When variables have been declared and options such as titles set then click OK. The resulting bar chart is shown in Figure 6.7.

Interpretation

Of those who checked their breasts at least once a month, white women are the pre-dominant ethnic group. Black women are the dominant group of those who checked their breasts daily.

Categories in the variable currently selected (denoted by a solid blue line around the Cluster: set color box)

Drag the variable that the chart is going to be by in this box. In this example, ethnic group has been dragged to this position

This can be changed to Percentage if the Y-Axis is required to represent the percentage of the total

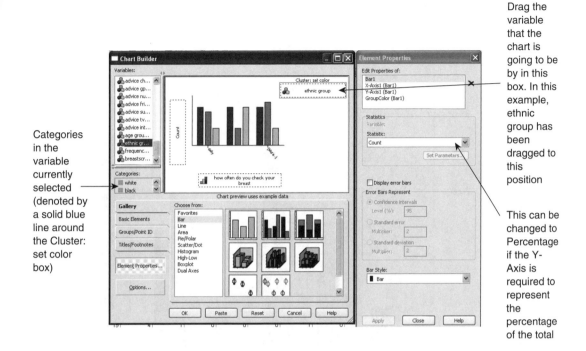

FIGURE 6.6   CHART BUILDER DIALOG BOX SHOWING CLUSTERED BAR CHART

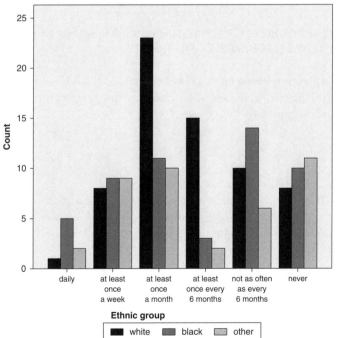

FIGURE 6.7   BAR CHART OF 'HOW OFTEN DO YOU CHECK YOUR BREASTS?' BY ETHNICITY

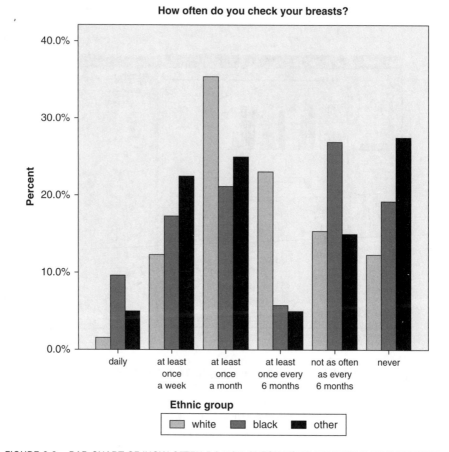

FIGURE 6.8   BAR CHART OF 'HOW OFTEN DO YOU CHECK YOUR BREASTS?' BY ETHNICITY WITH BARS EXPRESSED AS PERCENTAGE WITHIN ETHNICITY

Once again interpretation would be much easier if the bar chart showed percentages rather than counts. This can be requested by changing the Statistic: in the Element Properties dialog box (Figure 6.6).

Interpretation

Figure 6.8 shows the same data expressed as percentages within each ethnic group. It shows that more than 30% of white women check their breasts at least once a month but less than once a week. More than 20% of women from other ethnicities never check their breasts.

PIE CHARTS

A pie chart is used for showing the proportions (percentages) of an individual variable in a circular format, which looks similar to a pie. Whereby the larger the

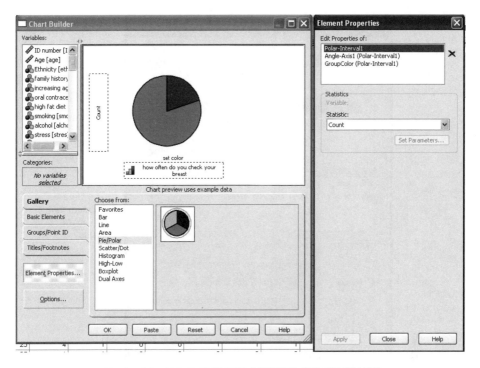

FIGURE 6.9   CHART BUILDER AND ELEMENT PROPERTIES FOR PIE CHARTS

slice of the pie, the greater the percentage (= number) of participants who fall into that given category. They can be constructed independently of the Frequencies… command described earlier in this chapter by clicking on Graphs → Chart Builder… and then selecting Pie/Polar from the list of possible chart types and dragging the pie chart picture to the large white box at the top of the Chart Builder dialog box, as shown in Figure 6.9. The variable of interest should be dragged to the Slice by? box (this has already done with the variable How often do you check your breasts? in Figure 6.9), the Angle Variable? box will then change to Count, this can be changed to Percentage by altering the Statistic: on the Element Properties part of the Chart Builder dialog box. When all attributes have been declared, click OK. The pie chart produced through these instructions looks the same as the one shown in Figure 6.2.

If the percentages or numbers that each slice represents is required to be shown on each slice, the pie chart constructed using the Chart Builder or Frequencies… can be edited using the Chart Editor, which is invoked by double clicking the relevant chart in SPSS Viewer. Once in the Chart Editor right click on the pie chart to give a number of options. Click on Properties Window to give the Properties dialog box shown in Figure 6.10. From this select the Data Value Labels tab. Move either the Percent or Count to the Displayed: box (Percent is the default, so Close can be clicked if that is the desired option, if anything else is selected, Apply should be clicked before Close). Whilst this dialog box is open, it is a good opportunity to edit other aspects of the pie chart. When all editing has been done, from the Chart Editor, click on File → Close to show the edited chart in SPSS Viewer.

Attributes that can be changed using this dialog box

Properties

| Chart Size | Text Layout | Text Style | Fill & Border |
| Number Format | | Data Value Labels | Variables |

Labels

Displayed:

Percent

The Data Value Label(s) that will be displayed

Not Displayed:

Count

how often do you check your breast

The Data Value Label(s) that will not be displayed

Label Position

○ Automatic

○ Manual

⊙ Custom

Use this box to alter where the labels appear

Display Options

☑ Suppress overlapping labels

☑ Display connecting lines to label

☐ Match label color to graphic element

Apply | Close | Help

SUMMARY

- Categorical variables should be summarised using frequencies. These show what percentage of responses fall into each category. In SPSS they can be generated using Analyze → Descriptive Statistics → Frequencies.... Where there are missing data, the Valid Percent in SPSS should be used. Valid Percent does not include missing data.
- Bar charts show categorical data graphically. Simple bar charts can be requested by clicking on Charts within Frequencies to request a bar chart. These can also be produced using the Chart Builder, whereby more complex bar charts can be produced.
- Pie charts also show categorical data graphically. These can be produced either by clicking on Charts within Frequencies to request a pie chart or they can also be generated using the Chart Builder.
- Both bar and pie charts can be edited using the Chart Editor to do such things as add additional labels and titles, edit existing labels and titles, change colour schemes and transpose the chart.

EXERCISES

TABLE 6.1   EPIDEMIOLOGICAL AND RISK FACTOR DATA FOR
2495 CULTURE POSITIVE TUBERCULOSIS PATIENTS FROM
GREATER LONDON, 1 JULY 1995 TO 31 DECEMBER 1997

Variable	%	n/N
Age		
0–19	7.1	178/2495
20–34	39.0	972/2495
35–59	32.5	812/2495
60+	17.6	437/2495
Unknown	3.9	96/2495
Sex		
Male	57.4	1433/2495
Female	40.1	1001/2495
Unknown	2.4	61/2495
Birth in UK		
UK born	14.0	273/1951
Not UK born	57.3	1117/1951
Unknown	28.8	561/1951
Ethnic origin		
White	17.9	348/1947
Indian sub-continent	22.1	431/1947
Black Caribbean	2.9	56/1947
Black African	25.2	490/1947
Black other	1.7	33/1947
Other	9.4	182/1947
Unknown	20.9	407/1947

Source: Maguire et al., 2002: 618

1   Using the data shown in Table 6.1, calculate the valid percentages for age group, sex, country of birth and ethnicity (take unknown to be missing).
2   Why should valid percentages be used in preference to percentages from SPSS output?
3   What other modifications could be made to Table 6.1 to improve its clarity?

Open smoking.sav. This is a small dataset looking at participants' smoking habits and some issues related to smoking.
   Request frequency tables for smoking status 'smoker' and the perceived length of smokers' work breaks in comparison to non-smokers 'smokebrea' from SPSS.

4   How many participants gave valid responses to smoking status?
5   How many participants and what percentage were never smokers?
6   What percentage of participants thought that smokers' breaks were the same length as non-smokers?
7   Give a possible reason for the missing data in the variable 'smokebrea', what could have been done to ensure less missing data?

7
SAMPLES AND POPULATIONS

INTRODUCTION

Before a study can take place, participants have to be selected and recruited. For research to be as credible as possible the study population needs to represent the population it is characterising as closely as possible. This is not always easy because it is often difficult to identify those who are members of the population. When doing research, time and finances often have to be taken into consideration when selecting participants to take part in a study, although this should not compromise the integrity of the research.

This chapter will discuss what a population is and the type of data collection that is undertaken on populations before moving onto samples, and sampling strategies. This will include examples from the literature of studies that have used specific sampling strategies. Finally this chapter will explore the consequences of using samples as opposed to the population, and the statistics, namely standard error and confidence intervals that are produced as a result.

THE AIMS OF THIS CHAPTER ARE:

- To learn the difference between samples and populations.
- To show the types of sampling techniques available, and when it is appropriate to use a given technique.
- To discuss the statistical consequences of sampling.

POPULATIONS

A population is defined as all those in a given place at a given time. This implies that populations might be large. An example of a large population is all those living in the United Kingdom today. It also implies that because they are large, it may not be known what the exact population is; it would be impossible to count everybody in the United Kingdom every day. People are born, die and migrate into and out of national and regional populations every day. Although statistics representing these changes are collected, these do not represent changes on a day-to-day basis because the changes (such as birth or death registrations) are not always reported on the day they occur and migration is harder to quantify.

Other populations are smaller and may be easier to quantify, such as the number of people employed at a given institution, where the Human Resources department keeps records. The number of people in-patient in a given hospital on a specific date or the number with a specific condition is recorded by the hospital. However, like the national populations, these populations are also transient; in addition to birth, death and migration, in occupational populations, people can leave their job or become a new employee. In disease/hospital populations, people can become ill or recover from the illness.

CENSUS

Data collection from the whole population is called census. Most countries have had at least one census of the entire population. The United Kingdom and United States of America carries out censuses of the population every ten years, whilst Australia carries out its census every five years (ABS, 2007; ONS, 2007a; US Census Bureau, 2007). The United Kingdom population census collects information on demographics, student status, migration, ethnicity, identity and religion, health status, occupation and qualifications (ONS, 2007a). It is impossible to carry out the census more frequently because it is costly to undertake. Linked to that, it is also time consuming. The population census takes a lot of planning in terms of the questions to be asked (these are often piloted some time before the actual census) and the actual logistics of carrying out the census. Forms have to be delivered to all households. When the forms have been returned, data analysis takes years. An ongoing census occurs through birth and death registration of those who are born and died in the UK.

Smaller censuses may be in the form of how many people are in a hospital at a given time with a given condition or needing a given treatment. This type of information can be used for planning purposes so that, for example it is known the number of dialysis machines that will be needed.

SAMPLES

Samples are groups of participants selected to make inferences about the populations from which they are drawn. For example Zhu et al.'s 2004 study included 1896 students in China, November 1994 to March 1995. This is a sample of students studying in China between November 1994 and March 1995. If a population is small, for example those with a rare disease, sampling may not be useful because the sample may be too small to make meaningful inferences and in these circumstances it may be possible to do a census as easily as sampling. Samples are taken to reduce the time it would take to carry out the study if the population was used. In addition, taking a sample decreases the costs of the study compared with studying the whole population.

To be able to make accurate inferences about the population the sample should be representative of the population from which it is drawn. For example, taking a sample of people in hospital is not representative of people who live in a given town or country. These people will have a worse health status and are likely to be older on average than the general population of a town.

Another potential problem that should be considered in relation to taking samples is the issue of bias. Bias can occur in a number of ways, including as a result of choosing a sample that is not representative of the population in question. Even if the plan is to select a sample that is representative of the population in question, biases can still occur. For example, respondents may have different characteristics to non-respondents. However, this may not be explicitly known during data collection because it is unlikely to be possible to gain baseline characteristics on those who do not respond.

Taking a random sample from the whole population ensures that the sample is representative of that population. Sampling strategies are discussed in the next section of this chapter. Sampling can still be a large task.

Simple random sampling

With simple random sampling, all members of the population have an equal probability of being a member of the sample. For this to occur it must be known who is in the population; a list of the members of the population is known as the sampling frame. As discussed earlier, populations are often large, which has implications for sampling, potentially making it a big job, both finding a complete and up-to-date sampling frame and subsequently numbering it. The sampling frame might be the electoral register if persons aged 18 or over are required, postcode address file if addresses are required, alternately it may be possible to obtain GP registers. All of these potential sampling frames have their problems which the researcher should be aware of, and where possible minimise possible biases. This way, if any biases occur in the study, they do so by chance. For example, bias may occur if research is via a telephone survey. This is biased against those who do not have telephones or whose telephone number is not listed in the telephone directory. Likewise, the fact that virtually any sampling frame employed will be out of date may be a potential source of bias.

Once a sampling frame has been obtained, each member of the population must then be numbered so that it can be uniquely identified. Then the drawing of the sample can begin. This can be done in a number of ways such as pulling numbers from a bag (although not recommended for large samples), using random number tables (Kirkwood and Sterne, 2003) to select the numbers that will be included in the sample or using a computer program to generate a list of random numbers. This process continues until the desired sample size has been reached.

A number of studies conducted in Sweden have used the Swedish Annual Level of Living Survey (SALLS), carried out by Statistics Sweden. Respondents were selected at random from the whole population, meaning that because of the size of the studies and the random selection, results were representative of the population. For example, Öhlander et al. (2006) looked at the relationship between non-employment and smoking status in people aged 25 to 64 years in 1993 to 2000 (n = 30826). In another study, data from this survey conducted in 1982 to 1983 were used to discover whether there was a relationship between general health in 1990 to 1991 and cultural activity at both baseline (1982 to 1983) and follow up (1990 to 1991) (Johansson et al., 2001).

Multistage random sampling

Multistage random sampling has the advantage over simple random sampling of not needing such large sampling frames. It is carried out by considering a sampling unit larger than the individual, but smaller than the population. This may be electoral wards, Primary Care Trusts, hospitals, Local Education Authorities or schools. Once a random sample of these units has been selected, individuals within these units are selected by taking a random sample from the larger units. Whilst this method of sampling may be administratively simpler than simple random sampling, individuals do not have an equal probability of being part of the sample (the larger units that are sampled do), meaning that the sample may not be representative of the population it is aiming to characterise.

Example from the literature

In Palaniappan et al.'s 2001 paper participants were selected from five regions of Canada; the remote regions were not included because of the high costs associated with conducting face-to-face interviews in remote areas. From within each of these, four census divisions were randomly selected with a probability in proportion to the population. Therefore, those census divisions that had higher populations were more likely to be part of the sample. This may also have been due to costs. Within each census division, two subdivisions were randomly selected, then, within those two, enumeration districts were selected. Finally, a random sample of households was taken using the electronic telephone directory.

Cluster sampling

Cluster sampling involves taking a random sample of units larger than the individual; these are the clustering unit, for example a school or GP practice. However, many recent papers found when using the keywords 'cluster sampling' in Medline and Web of Science were from the developing world, with clusters consisting of, for example, villages, health districts or rural or urban areas of a state.

When clusters have been selected, all the individuals within the cluster are invited to participate in the research. As participants are all recruited from the same place they will be more like one another than if the sample was taken at random. This can be accounted for in data analysis.

Example from the literature

Thorpe et al. (2006) conducted a population based cross sectional study of residents of New York, USA to determine the prevalence of a number of health conditions. To do this, they sampled clusters using a number of stages. In the first stage, 144 segments of the city (approximately one block) were randomly selected from more than 21000 segments. In the second stage, a sample of households was randomly selected from the segments previously selected. Under normal cluster sampling, the questionnaires would have been administered to everyone who satisfied the inclusion criteria from the selected households. However, in this study, participants within households were randomly selected, with people in a household with more than one eligible person having a greater probability of selection than single person households. This reduced the potential number of households that needed to be visited.

Stratified random sampling

Stratified random sampling is used to ensure that a given number or percentage of participants with a given characteristic are included in the sample. To undertake this, groups that are required to have the same number in have to be established, for example, sex, age groups or ethnicity. Once this has been established, a random sample is taken from within these groups. It may be difficult to find a sampling frame that specifically corresponds to the groups of interest. For example, the electoral roll in the United Kingdom does not break down those registered by sex, and only indicates those who will be 18 in the forthcoming year and those aged over 70. Therefore a sampling frame containing this information would have to be located to undertake stratified random sampling by age and sex.

Example from the literature

In the paper by Lacey et al. (2007) General Practitioner databases from one District Health Authority were used as the sampling frame to look at associations between piecework, musculoskeletal pain, physical and mental health. A random sample of 10000 participants was then taken from within four age groups, so that each age group was equally represented. However, data were only used on those whose longest serving job over the past five years was also their current job because current health status was being associated with employment.

Non-random sampling

It is not always possible to carry out any form of random sampling. Three non-random sampling strategies are described in the next section.

Convenience sampling

Convenience sampling is common in student projects because of the limited resources available and the relatively few resources needed to carry it out. This type of sampling involves recruiting those who happen to be available at the time of data collection to the study. This includes data collection that is carried out via the internet, such that the questionnaire is placed on a webpage and people choose to participate in the research. The major drawback of this sampling technique is that the sample may not be representative of the population.

For example, Covic et al.'s 2007 study used convenience sampling to survey community opinions on childhood obesity. The researchers sampled people in a number of locations willing to take part in their survey. The fact that there were potential biases in the sample was acknowledged to be limitations of the study by stating that the sample contained more women with tertiary education than the population. The researchers probably would not have been aware of this before the data were analysed.

Quota sampling

Quota sampling is often used by market researchers to ensure that they get a mixture of people in their sample, without having to know who the people in the sample are or their characteristics in advance of data collection. This type of sampling is not random so is liable to potential biases, although it is not always possible to know what these are or the reasons why they have occurred.

The first step in quota sampling is to decide which characteristics are likely to affect the outcome. Then the distribution of the population in relation to those factors should be investigated so that sampling can occur in the same proportions of the population. Finally, data can be collected as laid down by the quota until all criteria have been fulfilled.

However, there are a number of weaknesses in this method of sample selection. The first is that it is hard to think of all possible classifications of potential participants, and if a large number of classifications are used, then it can be difficult to find participants who match the quota criteria. It is difficult to assess reliability of quota sampling and the sample it produces, the only way to do so is to repeat the survey using the same criteria and/or to know the characteristics of the population the sample is representing to determine whether they are similar.

Example from the literature

> As no statistics about the size or demographic composition of the Gypsy and Traveller population in England are available, the lack of a sampling frame rules out probabilistic sampling methods. Instead, we quota-sampled across accommodation types, sex, age and ethnic subgroups within the Gypsy and Traveller population, and compared them with a concurrent English-speaking non-Traveller sample, matched for age and sex. (Parry et al., 2007: 199)

The paper by Parry et al. (2007) shows that the reason why quota sampling was used was because there was not a sampling frame (list of individuals who were travellers) from which a random sample could be taken. Therefore it was decided to take quotas on 'accommodation types, sex, age and ethnic subgroups within the Gypsy and Traveller population'. It was calculated that the quota for each characteristic should be 83 participants. The numbers recruited in relation to each characteristic is shown in the total column of Table 7.1. It shows that, for sex and ethnicity there was recruitment in excess of the quota, however, this was necessary to ensure the quota was met in terms of the type of site travellers lived on.

TABLE 7.1   RECRUITMENT BY QUOTA VARIABLES

Gypsies and Travellers	Quota	Total
Sex		
Male	83	102
Female	83	191
Ethnicity		
English/Welsh	83	139
Irish	83	141
Other		13
Site		
Council	83	96
Private		33
Unauthorised	83	84
Housed	83	80

Source: reproduced from Table 1 in Parry et al., 2007: 200

Systematic sampling

As the name suggests, this is where there is some element of system in the sampling method. This means that there is not an equal probability of all members of the population being in the sample implying that there are likely to be differences between the sample and the population. Therefore, any results gained from a study sampled in this way are unlikely to represent the population. An example of systematic sampling is selecting those who have an even year of birth, for example, 1928, 1956 or 1970.

Another method of systematic sampling is to invite potential participants to take part in a study if they appeared at given intervals in a list. For example, Paterson (1996) invited every seventh patient at her GP practice to take part in the research. Systematic sampling in this way is open to a lot of abuse, such that the people compiling the list can assign appointments that are not going to be part of the study to those who they do not want to be participants or vice versa. For example, they may choose not to assign appointments that would be part of the study to the elderly or children.

Therefore, this method of sampling should not be used when there are better alternatives to sampling which are more likely to give results that are applicable to the whole population.

In reality

In research, random sampling is not always possible because of a combination of the problems outlined in this chapter. Therefore samples often have to be taken from those available and willing to take part in the study. These are acknowledged as limitations of the study. The degree to which this occurs will impact on the generalisability of the study.

Consequences of sampling

Even when samples are drawn to represent the population, the results gained will not be exactly the same as those if results from the population were gained – there will be some random error. Likewise, if a study were repeated using the same population, but a different sample the statistics gained from the second study would differ from those of the first study. However, if a number of samples from the same population, measuring the same outcome were selected, these means would form a Normal distribution, and they would have a mean close to the population mean and would equal the population mean if an infinite number of samples were taken.

However, taking a large number of samples in the course of one study is unrealistic. Therefore a statistical quantity representing the margin of error around a sample is required. This is called the standard error (SE). The formula of the standard error includes the sample size, meaning that standard errors are smaller with larger sample sizes. The standard error is rarely reported when doing unifactorial statistical tests (Chapter 9), but may be reported when reporting the results of statistical modelling (Chapter 11).

95% Confidence intervals

Although standard errors are not usually reported following statistical analysis, they are a useful quantity used in the formulation of 95% confidence intervals (CI). Ninety-five percent confidence intervals are therefore linked to the issue of sampling because the smaller the sample, the more variation there is likely to be within the data and therefore the larger the standard error and the wider the 95% confidence interval, and vice versa.

The 95% confidence interval is the range of values of a given variable such that we can be 95% certain that the true population mean lies within the lower and upper confidence limits. Therefore the true population mean will lie outside the 95% confidence interval on one in 20 (5%) occasions. Apart from means, 95% CI can be calculated around percentages, differences in means, relative risks and odds ratios. It is good practice to present 95% CIs so that the reader can see how wide they are. When presenting 95% CI in the context of statistical tests or statistical models like the ones described later in this book, they indicate whether the result is statistically significant. That is, if calculating the difference between two means, statistical significance has been attained if the 95% CI does not cross the point of no difference; which would be 0.

Confidence intervals can be calculated for widths other than 95% (although 95% is the norm) such as 90% or 99%. If the confidence interval calculated is 90%, this will be narrower than a 95% confidence interval, and likewise if it is 99%, it will be wider than a 95% confidence interval.

For further information on the calculation of standard errors and 95% confidence intervals see Kirkwood and Sterne (2003).

SUMMARY

- Populations are often large, so it may not be possible to use them as a whole for research purposes.
- Samples can be used to do research on a smaller number of participants than the whole population. There are a number of possible methods for drawing samples. The most appropriate one for the research question and study design should be used.
- The statistics produced will not be the true population statistics (mean or percentage), so 95% confidence intervals should be shown where possible so that it can be shown within which limits the true population statistics are likely to lie.

EXERCISES

Using the information from published research papers below, answer the related questions.

TABLE 7.2   CROSSTABULATION OF AGE GROUP AND PIECEWORK WORKING STATUS

	Piecework		No piecework		p-value
Age	n/N	%	n/N	%	
18–44	44/201	22	303/992	31	0.010
45–54	80/201	40	382/992	38	
55–64	68/201	34	272/992	27	
65–75	9/201	4	35/992	4	

1 Using Table 7.2 giving the numbers and percentages doing piecework by age group in the UK (Lacey et al., 2007), what do you observe from this?
2 If you were to carry out the study, how would you change the stratified random sampling?

First, the investigators randomly selected 15 or 30 half days of consultation for each participating physician (depending on whether he/she worked part or full time). Next, each physician was asked to enrol every tenth worker undergoing a regularly scheduled annual health examination into the study. Thus, physicians followed a standardised random selection procedure, and were not able to choose study participants. (Melchior et al., 2006: 754).

3 Why is this not a random sample of French workers?
4 Give possible reasons for the study being designed in such a way.
5 How could the study design have been improved to ensure random selection of study participants?

Females vocalised 53% more words than males (mean 51 vs 33 respectively, 95% CI for the difference 11.4–24.2). (Marston et al., 2007: 593)

6 What is the difference in the mean number of words vocalised between females and males?
7 What does the 95% confidence interval indicate?

8
COMPARING TWO CATEGORICAL VARIABLES

INTRODUCTION

Many variables from health surveys and questionnaires produce categorical data such as gender, age group or smoking status. Initial analysis using frequencies as in Chapter 6 should be the starting point with this type of data. Following that, the simplest analyses of these is to determine how many participants and what percentage fall into the groups created by the two variables.

Once an analysis plan has been established, then significance tests can be set up. This chapter will explain the general process involved in setting up significance tests. Where one variable is the outcome (for example survival status, died versus survived) and the other is a possible explanatory variable (for example gender, male versus female) then the most appropriate test (ignoring external variables, which will be explored in Chapter 12) is the chi-square test or Fisher's exact test depending on whether the assumptions of the chi-square test have been met. Depending on the study design, it is often useful to present statistics to quantify the difference between the two groups. This can be done using risks and relative risks.

Cohen's Kappa can be used to quantify the level of agreement between two or more assessors who are assessing the same participants using the same criteria. Alternately (with care), kappa can be used to see whether participants have the same opinions or beliefs when assessed at two or more time points.

Finally, this chapter explains sensitivity and specificity; used in determining what percentage of the time a screening test for a given condition/disease gives the same diagnosis as the gold standard for diagnosing that condition/disease. This will be extended to show how cut-offs can be established by maximising sensitivity and specificity. This will be shown visually using ROC curves.

This chapter will be illustrated using a number of datasets. The first is a study of younger (18–49 years old) women staff working at a university and women students' knowledge of and attitudes to breast cancer. It will also use a workplace study of back pain. The final dataset that will be used in this chapter comes from a physiotherapy setting, where the mobility of a group of older people was assessed and related to their falls status.

THE AIMS OF THIS CHAPTER ARE:

- To crosstabulate two categorical variables.
- To discover whether there is a statistically significant association between two variables that are crosstabulated using the appropriate tests.
- To calculate risks and relative risks to quantify the difference between two groups.
- To determine whether there is more agreement than would be expected by chance between two assessors using Cohen's Kappa.
- To explain the concepts of sensitivity, specificity, positive predictive value, negative predictive value and ROC.
- To describe what these concepts aim to find out, when they are used and how to conduct and interpret them.

PRELIMINARIES TO THIS CHAPTER

$\sqrt{}$ is used to indicate that the quantity under the sign should be square rooted.

$\log_e$ is used to indicate taking logarithms to base e. On a scientific calculator this is shown as ln (and Ln in SPSS).

Antilogging (exponentiation) is done using the e^x key on a scientific calculator, and with Exp in SPSS.

CROSSTABULATIONS (SOMETIMES CALLED CONTINGENCY TABLES)

When checking data, crosstabulations can be useful for conducting logic checks; that is making sure that the answers in one variable are possible given the response to another variable. For example, making sure males have not answered yes to 'Are you currently pregnant?' because it is not possible for a male to be pregnant, so this question should not have been asked to males and the response should be missing because the question was not applicable.

Crosstabulations are the result of looking at two categorical variables to see how many participants (and what percentage of the study population) in a given group have a given characteristic. For example, what percentage of white women in a study are aware that increasing age is a risk factor for breast cancer.

To invoke crosstabulations in SPSS, click on Analyze → Descriptive Statistics → Crosstabs ... to give the dialog box shown in Figure 8.1.

Transfer one categorical variable to the Row(s): box and another categorical variable to the Column(s): box. The variables can be placed in the boxes in either order; the resulting table will convey the same information regardless of which way round the variables are shown in the crosstabulation. However, for presentation purposes it is conventional that the grouping variable is shown in the columns and the disease/condition or exposure is shown in the rows. In this example age group has been placed in the columns and whether participants think increasing age is a risk factor for breast cancer has been placed in the rows.

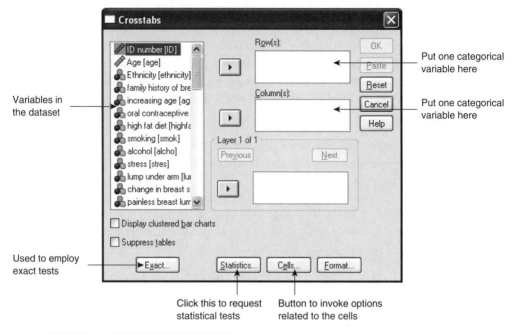

FIGURE 8.1   CROSSTABS DIALOG BOX

When the variables have been declared, click on the Cells ... button to add additional information regarding each cell (Figure 8.2). From this dialog box, tick Row and Column percentages. When options relating to cells have been selected, click Continue to return to the Crosstabs dialog box (Figure 8.1). Then click OK to get the output shown in Figure 8.3.

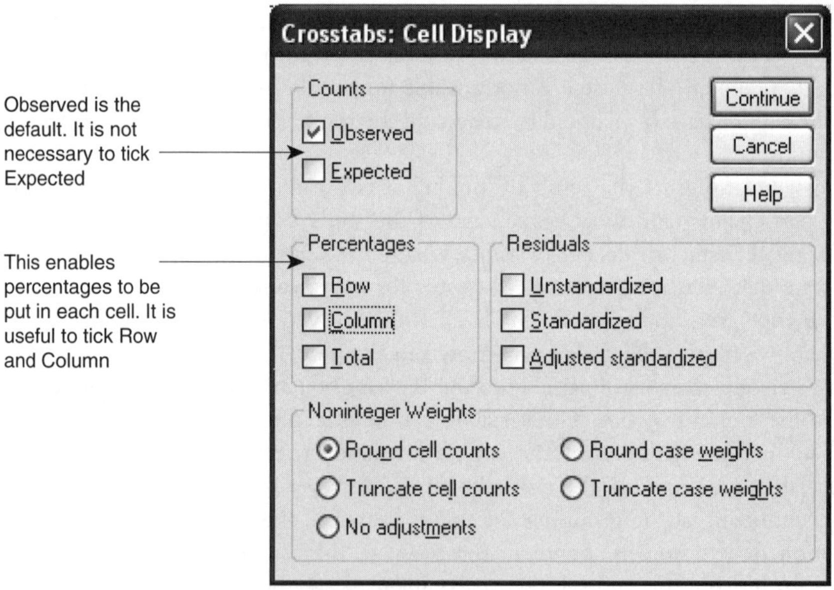

FIGURE 8.2   CROSSTABS: CELL DISPLAY DIALOG BOX

Case Processing Summary

	Cases						Number of respondents who were not aware that increasing age was a risk factor for breast cancer
	Valid		Missing		Total		
	N	Percent	N	Percent	N	Percent	
Increasing age * age group	157	96.9%	5	3.1%	162	100.0%	

Increasing age * age group Crosstabulation

			Age group					
			18–24	25–34	35–44	45–49	Total	
Increasing age	no	Count	66	30	17	11	(124)	
		% within increasing age	53.2%	24.2%	13.7%	8.9%	100.0%	
		% within age group	90.4%	73.2%	63.0%	68.8%	79.0%	
	yes	Count	7	11	10	5	33	
		% within increasing age	21.2%	(33.3%)	30.3%	15.2%	100.0%	
		% within age group	9.6%	26.8%	37.0%	(31.2%)	21.0%	
Total		Count	(73)	41	27	16	(157)	Total number of respondents
		% within increasing age	46.5%	26.1%	17.2%	10.2%	100.0%	
		% within age group	100.0%	100.0%	100.0%	100.0%	100.0%	

Number of respondents aged 18 to 24 years

Of those who thought increasing age was a risk factor for breast cancer, 33% were aged 25 to 34 years

Of those who were aged 45 to 49, 31% thought that increasing age was a risk factor for breast cancer

FIGURE 8.3   AGE GROUP VERSUS WHETHER WOMEN ARE AWARE THAT INCREASING AGE IS A RISK FACTOR FOR BREAST CANCER

The Case Processing Summary shows that there were five respondents that did not answer one or both questions that comprise this crosstabulation, so were not included in this analysis.

In this study, age group was the grouping variable and knowledge of increasing age as a risk factor for breast cancer was the exposure variable.

Interpretation

Ten percent (7/73) of 18 to 24 year olds were aware that increasing age was a risk factor for breast cancer. The percentage of women who were aware of increasing age being a risk factor for breast cancer increased with increasing age to those in the 35 to 44 years old age group at 37% (10/27) before decreasing to 31% in those aged 45 to 49 years (5/16).

Note: SPSS output tables such as Figure 8.3 should not be placed in final reports, dissertations or theses. The required information should be selected and put in the text as shown with the interpretation and/or put in a table if there are a number of results from the same study. An example of how to do this is given in Peacock and Kerry (2007).

HYPOTHESIS TESTING

Before a hypothesis can be set up or tested, the question of what a hypothesis is needs to be addressed. In this context, it is an untested statement about relationships or associations between factors. Hypotheses are set up so that they can be tested using significance tests to determine whether there is an association between the factors in question. Before a significance test can be carried out, two hypotheses have to be set up; these are called the null hypothesis (denoted H_0) and the alternative hypothesis (denoted H_1 or H_A). These take the general form:

> H_0: There is no difference in the population from which the sample is drawn between the two groups on the variable being tested.
> H_1: There is a difference in the population from which the sample is drawn between the two groups on the variable being tested.

The null hypothesis is always a hypothesis of no difference between groups. Notice these hypotheses are open to the possibility of any difference between the variables in question and does not specify which way any differences may occur. This is called setting up a two sided hypothesis. It is usual to set up a two sided hypotheses in health and medical research. A one sided hypothesis gives an alternative of the form:

> H_1: Group 1 is higher (better) than group 2 in the population that the sample is taken.

A good, justifiable, a priori reason should be given in the methods section of the report, dissertation, thesis or paper for using one sided tests because they ignore any differences that may occur in the other direction.

When null and alternative hypotheses have been set up, an appropriate test can be run, and the weight of evidence against the null hypothesis can be assessed with the p-value. The meaning of p-values was explained in Chapter 4.

CHI-SQUARE TEST

Chi-square tests (also written as χ^2, χ is the Greek letter chi) are used to see whether there is a relationship between two categorical variables by comparing the proportions (percentages) in each cell. Any size of crosstabulation from two by two (two categorical variables, both with two categories) upwards can be used. For example, the crosstabulation used in Figure 8.3 was a four by two table because age group had four categories and awareness of increasing age as a risk factor for breast cancer had two categories. The chi-square test is used for large samples, and has the assumptions that 80% of cells have an expected count of greater than five and all cells have an expected count of greater than one. The expected count is generated in the calculation of the chi-square test. It is not necessary for the concept of expected counts to be understood for the chi-square test to be understood (although SPSS will display expected counts if requested by ticking the appropriate box in the Crosstabs: Cell Display dialog box, shown in Figure 8.2). SPSS gives a footnote after computing the chi-square test to indicate whether the assumptions of this test have been violated.

Before a test can be carried out, null and alternative hypotheses have to be set up. Using the same variables as for the crosstabulations example, these are:

H_0: There is no difference in the awareness of increasing age as a risk factor for breast cancer between women in increasing age groups aged 18 to 49 years.

H_1: There is a difference in the awareness of increasing age as a risk factor for breast cancer between women in increasing age groups aged 18 to 49 years.

To do a chi-square test in SPSS, open the Crosstabs dialog box (Figure 8.1) as previously described in the section on crosstabulations earlier in this chapter, and select the variables for the Rows: and Columns: boxes. From the Crosstabs: Cell Display dialog box (Figure 8.2), choose Row and Column percentages, then click Continue to return to the Crosstabs dialog box (Figure 8.1). Click the Statistics ... button to get the Crosstabs: Statistics dialog box shown in Figure 8.4.

Select Chi-square then click Continue to return to the Crosstabs dialog box (Figure 8.1), then click OK. In addition to the output shown in Figure 8.3, the results of the chi-square test are also produced. These are shown in Figure 8.5 (the Case Processing Summary and Crosstabulation have been suppressed).

The footnote in Figure 8.5 indicates that the assumptions of the chi-square test have not been violated as only 12.5% (1 cell of 8) of cells had an expected count of less than five, so the test is valid. If this was more than 20% then the chi-square test would not be valid. The Value of 11.760 is the Chi-square test statistic for this test; this derives from calculations using the observed and expected values. The level of significance of this value depends on the degrees of freedom (df), which is shown in the next column. In this test there are three degrees of freedom. This derives from (number of columns−1) $\times$ (number of rows−1), giving $(4-1) \times (2-1) = 3$. In health journals there is no longer emphasis on reporting the test statistic and degrees of freedom and a move towards reporting the percentages and the p-value. The p-value

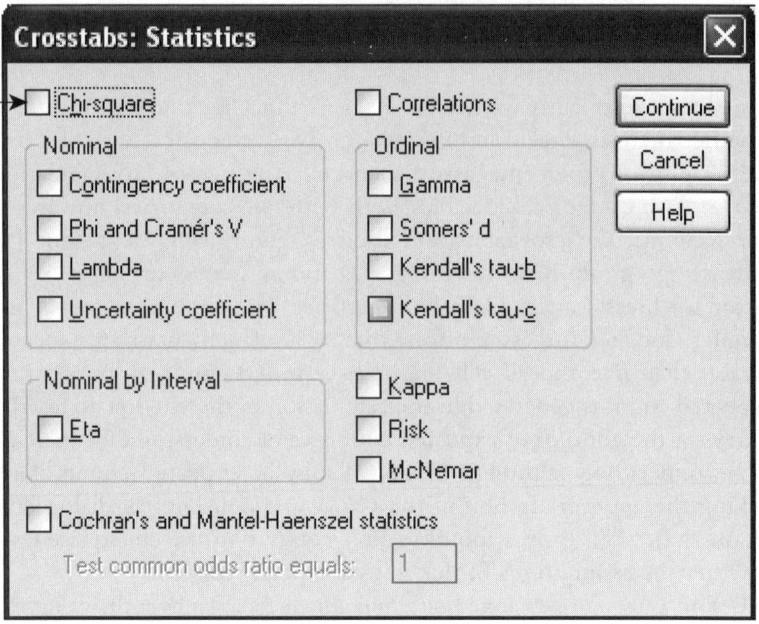

Tick this box to request Chi-square test

FIGURE 8.4   CROSSTABS: STATISTICS DIALOG BOX

Chi-Square Tests

	Values	df	Asymp. Sig. (2-sided)
Pearson Chi-Square	11.760[a]	3	.008
Likelihood Ratio	12.176	3	.007
Linear-by-Linear Association	9.347	1	.002
N of Valid Cases	157		

The relevant data pertaining to the chi-square test is found on the top line of this table

[a] 1 cells (12.5%) have expected count less than 5. The minimum expected count is 3.36.

FIGURE 8.5   CHI-SQUARE TEST OUTPUT FOR AGE GROUP VERSUS WHETHER WOMEN ARE AWARE THAT INCREASING AGE IS A RISK FACTOR FOR BREAST CANCER

for the chi–square test is shown on the Pearson Chi–Square row of Figure 8.5 in the Asymp. Sig. (2-sided) column.

Interpretation

Ten percent (7/73) of 18 to 24 year olds were aware that increasing age was a risk factor for breast cancer. The percentage of women who were aware of increasing age being a risk factor for breast cancer increased with increasing age to those in the 35 to 44 years old age group at 37% (10/27) before decreasing to 31% in those aged 45 to 49 years (5/16). This was highly significant (p = 0.008), indicating a relationship between age of women in the survey and their knowledge of whether increasing age is a risk factor for breast cancer.

IF ASSUMPTIONS OF THE CHI-SQUARE TEST ARE VIOLATED

Collapsing categories

If the assumptions of the chi-square test do not hold it may be possible to collapse some categories to give fewer cells with larger cell counts. For example, looking at the data shown in Figures 8.3 and 8.5, the age groups could be collapsed to make fewer of them, which in a crosstabulation would give fewer cells. This can be done using Recode in SPSS (See Chapter 2). Common sense should prevail when recoding such data, for example, only two adjacent age groups should be combined. For example, it would be permissible to combine age groups 35 to 44 and 45 to 49. However, it would be illogical to combine age groups 18 to 24 with 45 to 49 because it would be difficult to draw inferences.

Fisher's exact test

Fisher's exact test can be used as an alternative to collapsing categories when the assumptions of the chi-square test have been violated. For example, if the study demands that all groups are preserved, groups are so unique that it is not possible to combine two or more categories or the variables are already both two categories. Fisher's exact test does not have any assumptions that have to be adhered to. Where the crosstabulation is 2 by 2 (the variables in the rows and columns both have two categories), the p-value for Fisher's exact test is automatically calculated when the chi-square test has been requested. However, where the crosstabulation is larger, for example four columns and two rows, Fisher's exact test has to be specifically requested using the dialog box in Figure 8.6.

To invoke Fisher's exact test in SPSS, click on Analyze → Descriptive Statistics → Crosstabs…. This will give the Crosstabs dialog box (Figure 8.1), as with crosstabulations and the chi-square test. Move appropriate categorical variable to the Row(s) and Column(s) boxes. Request row and column percentages from the Crosstabs: Cell Display dialog box (Figure 8.2). Tick Chi-Square in the Crosstabs: Statistics dialog box (Figure 8.4). Finally, on the Crosstabs dialog box, click the Exact … button to give the dialog box shown in Figure 8.6.

On the Exact Tests dialog box (Figure 8.6), click the Exact radio button, then click Continue to return to the Crosstabs dialog box (Figure 8.1) then click OK to give the output shown in Figure 8.7. The p-value for Fisher's exact test is shown in the row labelled Fisher's Exact Test, in the column labelled Exact Sig. (2-sided). Where the crosstabulation is large (many rows and columns), Fisher's exact test may take a long time to calculate and occasionally it may not be possible for SPSS to calculate Fisher's exact test.

This example output is from the same breast cancer awareness dataset. In this example, the relationship between age group and knowledge of whether a lump under the arm is a symptom of breast cancer is examined.

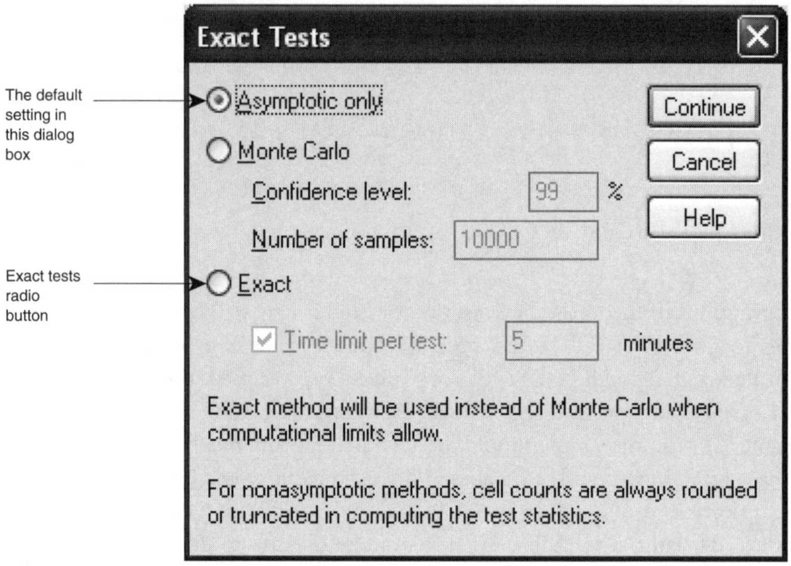

The default setting in this dialog box

Exact tests radio button

FIGURE 8.6   EXACT TESTS DIALOG BOX

The footnote in Figure 8.7 indicates that the assumptions of the chi-square test have been violated because more than 20% of cells have an expected count less than five; therefore, Fisher's exact test should be used.

Interpretation

Awareness of a lump under the arm as a symptom of breast cancer was high. Eighty-eight percent of women aged 25 to 34 years old (36/41) were aware of a lump under the arm being a symptom of breast cancer. The age group that was least aware of a lump under the arm being a symptom of breast cancer was those aged 44 to 49 years old at 75% (12/16). This was not statistically significant (p = 0.636).

RISK

Although the chi-square test provide us with a p-value to indicate whether a relationship between variables is significant (or not), it is unable to quantify the effect size. Therefore, there are a number of ways of quantifying these to show how different the proportions are. These all utilise two by two tables, but can be extended to other sizes of tables by using one category as the baseline category to compare with other categories.

Risk is mostly used in the context of prospective studies. It is the proportion of participants in a given population, initially free of a disease or condition who develop it within a specified time (usually defined by the bounds of the study). Risk does not have any time limits, but its value increases with increasing follow-up time.

Case Processing Summary

	Cases					
	Valid		Missing		Total	
	N	Percent	N	Percent	N	Percent
lump under arm *age group	157	96.9%	5	3.1%	162	100.0%

Lump under arm * age group Crosstabulation

			Age group				
			18–24	25–34	35–44	45–49	Total
lump under arm	no	Count	14	5	4	4	27
		% within lump under arm	51.9%	18.5%	14.8%	14.8%	100.0%
		% within age group	19.2%	12.2%	14.8%	25.0%	17.2%
	yes	Count	59	36	23	12	130
		% within lump under arm	45.4%	27.7%	17.7%	9.2%	100.0%
		% within age group	80.8%	87.8%	85.2%	75.0%	82.8%
Total		Count	73	41	27	16	157
		% within lump under arm	46.5%	26.1%	17.2%	10.2%	100.0%
		% within age group	100.0%	100.0%	100.0%	100.0%	100.0%

Chi-Square Tests

	Value	df	Asymp. Sig. (2-sided)	Exact Sig. (2-sided)	Exact Sig. (1-sided)	Point Probability
Pearson Chi-Square	1.713[a]	3	.634	.643		
Likelihood Ratio	1.711	3	.634	.655		
Fisher's Exact Test	1.793			.636		
Linear-by-Linear Association	.007[b]	1	.933	1.000	.500	.081
N of Valid Cases	157					

The Fisher's exact test p-value

[a] 2 cells (25.0%) have expected count less than 5. The minimum expected count is 2.75.
[b] The standardized statistic is –.084.

FIGURE 8.7   FISHER'S EXACT TEST OUTPUT FOR AGE GROUP VERSUS WHETHER WOMEN ARE AWARE THAT A LUMP UNDER THE ARM IS A SYMPTOM OF BREAST CANCER

Case Processing Summary

	Cases					
	Valid		Missing		Total	
	N	Percent	N	Percent	N	Percent
Lower Back pain * Is your job stressful?	211	79.0%	56	21.0%	267	100.0%

Lower Back pain * is your job stressful? Crosstabulation

			Is your job stressful?		
			stress free	stressful	Total
Lower Back pain	NoLBP	Count	96	44	140
		% within Lower Back pain	68.6	31.4	100.0%
		% within Is your job stressful?	73.8%	54.3%	66.4%
	LBP	Count	34	37	71
		% within Lower Back pain	47.9%	52.1%	100.0%
		% within Is your job stressful?	26.2%	45.7%	33.6%
Total		Count	130	81	211
		% within Lower Back pain	61.6	38.4%	100.0%
		% within Is your job stressful?	100.0%	100.0%	100.0%

Chi-Square Tests

	Value	df	Asymp. Sig. (2-sided)	Exact Sig. (2-sided)	Exact Sig. (1-sided)
Pearson Chi-Square	8.521[b]	1	.004		
Continuity Correction[a]	7.669	1	.006		
Likelihood Ratio	8.428	1	.004		
Fisher's Exact Test				.004	.003
Linear-by-Linear Association	8.481	1	.004		
N of Valid Cases	211				

[a]Computed only for a 2×2 table.
[b]0 cells (.0%) have expected count less than 5. The minimum expected count is 27. 26.

FIGURE 8.8   CROSSTABULATION OF LOWER BACK PAIN BY STRESSFUL JOB STATUS

This is intuitive since in a cohort study participants are followed and it is inevitable that more will get the disease or condition of interest with increasing time.

The example given in Figure 8.8 is from the workplace study of back pain. It shows a crosstabulation and chi–square test of whether the job is stressful versus lower back pain.

Interpretation

Thirty-four percent of participants (71/211) had Lower Back pain. Forty-six percent of those with a stressful job had Lower Back pain, whilst 26% of those without a stressful job had Lower Back pain. This was statistically significant p = 0.004.

Risk difference

The simplest way of examining risk and quantifying differences in proportions for presenting with a chi-square test p-value is to take the difference in proportions between the groups. This is called the risk difference. Using the data shown in Figure 8.8, the proportion of people with a stressful job with Lower Back pain is 37/81 = 0.457 and the proportion of people without a stressful job with Lower Back pain is 34/130 = 0.262. The risk difference of Lower Back pain for those with a stressful job minus those without a stressful job is 0.457 − 0.262 = 0.195 (19.5%). The chi-square test shown in Figure 8.8 shows that this difference in proportions is significant (p = 0.004). It is possible to calculate 95% confidence intervals around risk differences. A 95% CI for a risk difference that contains 0 (the null value) indicates that the difference in proportions is not statistically significant. SPSS does not calculate the risk difference or associated 95% confidence interval.

Calculating the 95% confidence interval for the risk difference

The key to calculating the 95% CI for the risk difference is the calculation of the standard error (SE) for the difference. This is calculated using the formula shown in Figure 8.9. p_1 and p_2 are the proportions in the first group and second groups respectively. n_1 and n_2 are the total numbers in groups 1 and 2 respectively. In relation to the output shown in Figure 8.8, the proportion in group 1 (p_1), which relates to those with a stressful job is 0.457; calculated from 37/81, meaning that $1 - p_1$ is $1 - 0.457 = 0.543$, and n_1 is 81 (the total number of people with a stressful job in the dataset). Likewise, the proportion in group 2 (p_2), representing those without a stressful job is 0.262 (34/130); $1 - p_2$ is $1 - 0.262 = 0.738$, and n_2 is 130 (the total number of people without a stressful job in the dataset). These can be placed into the formula shown in Figure 8.9 to give the worked example shown in Figure 8.10.

$$SE = \sqrt{\frac{p_1(1-p_1)}{n_1} + \frac{p_2(1-p_2)}{n_2}}$$

FIGURE 8.9   FORMULA FOR THE STANDARD ERROR OF A RISK DIFFERENCE

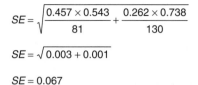

$$SE = \sqrt{\frac{0.457 \times 0.543}{81} + \frac{0.262 \times 0.738}{130}}$$

$$SE = \sqrt{0.003 + 0.001}$$

$$SE = 0.067$$

FIGURE 8.10   WORKED EXAMPLE OF THE CALCULATION OF THE STANDARD ERROR FOR A RISK DIFFERENCE

The 95% confidence interval for the difference can now be calculated using the formula: Risk difference ± (1.96 × standard error for the difference). The lower 95% confidence limit is $0.195 - (1.96 \times 0.067) = 0.063$, whilst the upper 95% confidence limit is $0.195 + (1.96 \times 0.067) = 0.327$.

Note: When calculating the SE and 95% confidence interval all decimal places given on the calculator have been retained, so calculations using the proportions shown in Figure 8.10 may differ slightly to those presented in the interpretation.

Interpretation

The difference in risk between those with and without a stressful job was 0.195, (95% CI 0.063, 0.327). The 95% confidence interval indicates 95% confidence that the true population difference in risk may be as small as 0.063 or as large as 0.327. As the 95% confidence interval does not cross 0 (the null value), it indicates, that this difference is statistically significant.

Relative risk

Relative risk (RR) is best explained using the schematic diagram shown in Table 8.1. This shows the data divided into two groups, which could be those exposed to a given condition such as a workplace chemical versus those not exposed. Groups could also represent smokers and non-smokers or gender. Risk for group 1 is calculated as a/(a+c) and risk for group 2 is calculated as b/(b+d). Using the data in Figure 8.8, the risk of Lower Back pain for those with a stressful job is $37/81 = 0.457$ and the risk of Lower Back pain for those without a stressful job is $34/130 = 0.262$. Note: because of the coding in SPSS, the data in Figure 8.8 are inverted compared to Table 8.1.

TABLE 8.1   SCHEMATIC DIAGRAM OUTLINING A CROSSTABULATION TO CALCULATE RISK AND RELATIVE RISK

		Group 1	Group 2	Total
Disease or condition of interest	Present	a	b	a+b
	Absent	c	d	c+d
	Total	a+c	b+d	a+b+c+d

Relative risk can be calculated using the formula: (a/(a+c))/(b/(b+d)). Using the data shown in Figure 8.8 the relative risk of Lower Back pain (those with a stressful job/those without a stressful job) is 0.457/0.262 = 1.75. SPSS does not calculate relative risk or its associated 95% confidence interval.

If the relative risk = 1 (the null value), then the risk in group 1 is the same as the risk in group 2, and no association between the two groups has been shown.

If the relative risk is <1 (less than 1) the risk in group 1 is less than the risk in group 2. This is a negative association, which may be protective.

If the relative risk is >1 (greater than 1) the risk in group 2 is greater than the risk in group 2. This is a positive association, which may be adverse.

Calculating the 95% confidence interval for the relative risk

As with calculating the 95% confidence interval for the difference in risk, the key to computing the 95% confidence interval for the relative risk is the determination of the standard error. The standard error that is calculated relates to the logarithm to base e. The formula that is used is shown in Figure 8.11 using notation from Table 8.1. This is shown in practical terms using the data in Figure 8.8 as a worked example in Figure 8.12.

Before the 95% confidence limit for the RR can be calculated, the relative risk needs to be logged to base e because this will be used as the point estimate in the relative risk before it is antilogged (exponentiated) when the $\log_e$ 95% confidence interval has been calculated. It will then be on the same scale as the SE calculated in Figure 8.12. The 95% confidence interval for the $\log_e$ relative risk is calculated using a similar formula to previously, that is: $\log_e$ (relative risk) ± 1.96 (standard error of the $\log_e$ relative risk). Using the data shown in Figure 8.8, the relative risk is 1.75 (shown earlier in this chapter), meaning the $\log_e$ (relative risk) is 0.558. The lower confidence limit for the $\log_e$ relative risk is 0.558 − (1.96 × 0.191) = 0.184. The upper confidence limit for the $\log_e$ relative risk is 0.558 + (1.96 × 0.191) = 0.932.

$$SE(\log_e RR) = \sqrt{\left(\frac{1}{a} - \frac{1}{a+c}\right) + \left(\frac{1}{b} - \frac{1}{b+d}\right)}$$

FIGURE 8.11   FORMULA FOR THE STANDARD ERROR OF LOG$_e$ RELATIVE RISK

$$SE(\log_e RR) = \sqrt{\left(\frac{1}{37} - \frac{1}{81}\right) + \left(\frac{1}{34} - \frac{1}{130}\right)}$$

$$SE(\log_e RR) = \sqrt{(0.027 - 0.012) + (0.029 - 0.008)}$$

$$SE(\log_e RR) = 0.191$$

FIGURE 8.12   WORKED EXAMPLE OF THE CALCULATION OF THE STANDARD ERROR FOR LOG$_e$ RELATIVE RISK

For presentation these need to be converted to 95% confidence intervals for the relative risk calculated earlier. To do this the results achieved (0.184 and 0.932) need to be antilogged (exponentiated) giving a 95% confidence interval for the relative risk 1.75 (from the data in Figure 8.8) of 1.20, 2.54. If the 95% confidence interval includes 1 (the null value), this indicates that statistical significance has not been achieved.

Interpretation

In terms of the example shown in Figure 8.8, the relative risk of Lower Back pain in those with and without a stressful job is 1.75 (95% CI 1.20, 2.54). This is statistically significant.

COHEN'S KAPPA

Cohen's Kappa, sometimes called kappa, denoted by κ (Greek small kappa) is used to assess the extent of agreement between two (or more) assessors for a categorical outcome. The assessors can be two (or more) people who are measuring the same outcome using the same measure. Alternately, it could be used to determine whether there is agreement between the same individuals at different time points. If using kappa for the latter reason, ensure that measuring agreement over time is sensible. SPSS is only able to analyse data where there are two assessors (time points). As kappa is measuring agreement between two assessors assessing the same thing, it follows that the crosstabulation will have the same number of categories in the rows as in the columns (for example, developmentally delayed versus normal development); SPSS expects this and will not calculate kappa unless this is the case.

The value of kappa ranges between 0 and 1, where 0 is no greater agreement than would have occurred by chance between the two raters and 1 is perfect agreement between the raters. Levels of agreement are usually categorised as (Altman, 1991):

Value of Kappa	Strength of agreement
<0.20	Poor
0.21–0.40	Fair
0.41–0.60	Moderate
0.61–0.80	Good
0.81–1.00	Very good

Therefore, it is desirable to have a kappa statistic greater than 0.60. SPSS provides a p-value for kappa; however, this is not usually reported in papers, dissertations or theses since the null hypothesis of no association between the raters is not logical for this test.

Kappa is implemented in SPSS through the Crosstabs ... command (Analyze →
Descriptive Statistics → Crosstabs...) to give the Crosstabs dialog box (Figure 8.1).
From the Crosstabs: Statistics dialog box (Figure 8.4), tick Kappa (Chi-Square should
not be ticked). When all options have been selected, click OK on the Crosstabs dialog box to give the output.

The example used here is to show the agreement between two raters assessing cranial ultrasound scans from UKOS. Scans have been rated into two categories, normal versus abnormal (Figure 8.13).

Case Processing Summary

	Cases					
	Valid		Missing		Total	
	N	Percent	N	Percent	N	Percent
Rater 2 * Rater 1	325	40.8%	472	59.2%	797	100.0%

Rater 2 * Rater 1 Crosstabulation

Count

		Rater 1		Total
		Normal	Abnormal	
Rater 2	Normal	230	23	253
	Abnormal	21	51	72
Total		251	74	325

Symmetric Measures

	Value	Asymp. Std. Error[a]	Approx.[b]	Approx.Sig.
Measure of Agreement Kappa	.611	.053	11.023	.000
N of Valid Cases	325			

[a]Not assuming the null hypothesis.
[b]Using the asymptotic standard error assuming the null hypothesis.

FIGURE 8.13   COHEN'S KAPPA FOR UKOS CRANIAL ULTRASOUND SCAN RESULTS

Interpretation

Data were available for 325 participants. Looking at the Rater 2 * Rater 1
Crosstabulation, rater 1 evaluated 251 scans as normal and 74 as abnormal, whereas
rater 2 considered 253 scans to be normal and 72 to be abnormal. Where both rater
1 and rater 2 evaluated the scans as normal (n = 230) and where both raters judged
the scans to be abnormal (n = 51) there is agreement between the two raters. The off
diagonals, where one rater considers scans to be normal and the other one considers

them to be abnormal are where there is disagreement. Looking at the Symmetric Measures box (Figure 8.13), the kappa value is 0.611 indicating good agreement between the two raters.

It is most likely that the value of kappa would be reported in the text of a dissertation or thesis since it is not likely that a large number of kappa will be carried out on the same dataset. Output like Figure 8.13 should not be included.

SENSITIVITY AND SPECIFICITY

Within health and medical settings, diagnostic tests are carried out for virtually all conditions, for example the Bayley Scales of Infant Development (Bayley, 1993) can indicate whether a child has developmental delay and pathology is used to diagnose the presence of cancers. For example, when diagnosing cancer, often patients have a scan (for example an MRI) before they have a more invasive test such as a biopsy. The results from these two tests can be crosstabulated to show the relationship between the results of the two tests. An example of the relationship between a liver scan and liver pathology can be seen in Altman and Bland (1994).

For statistical analysis to take place, one of the diagnostic tests needs to be established as the 'gold standard' or 'criterion test'. This means the test that is considered to be definitive. Of course the definitive test can change over time as technology and other factors change. In Altman and Bland's 1994 example liver pathology was the 'gold standard' and a liver scan is the test.

From the crosstabulation a number of statistics can be calculated to describe the relationship between the two tests. The first is sensitivity, defined as the proportion of test positives that are true positives (where test refers to the screening test and true refers to the result gained on the 'gold standard' test). The second is specificity, defined as the proportion of test negatives that are also true negatives. These can either be expressed as a proportion or a percentage. SPSS does not explicitly calculate sensitivity and specificity, although they can be elicited fairly easily by correct extraction of crosstabulation percentages.

The worked example in this chapter uses falls status in older people (whether they have had recurrent falls) as the gold standard because it is known whether the participants have fallen more than once. The screening test, Performance Oriented Assessment of Mobility (POAM) (Tinetti, 1986) assesses balance and gait. Using the data presented here a cut-off of 20 (those who scored <20 versus those who scored 20 or more) on the POAM was found to be the best at differentiating between those who were recurrent fallers and those who were not. These are shown in the crosstabulation in Figure 8.14.

Interpretation

From the crosstabulation shown in Figure 8.14 some important quantities are seen. The first quantity is the prevalence of recurrent falls in this study population. In this example it is 32/50 = 0.64 (64%). This is the total number who are true positives divided by the total number in the study. Next is sensitivity, which is 24/32 = 0.75

POAM with a cut off of 20 * Falls Status Crosstabulation

			Falls Status		
			Not fallen recurrently	Fallen recurrently	Total
POAM with a cut off of 20	Not at risk of recurrent falling	Count % within Falls Status	15 83.3%	8 25.0%	23 46.0%
	At risk of recurrent falling	Count % within Falls Status	3 16.7%	24 75.0%	27 54.0%
Total		Count % within Falls Status	18 100.0%	32 100.0%	50 100.0%

The number who are true negative and test negative. The percentage of true negatives that are also test negative (specificity)

The number who are true positive and test positive. The percentage of true positives that are also test positive (sensitivity)

FIGURE 8.14   CROSSTABULATION OF RECURRENT FALLS STATUS AND POAM SHOWING SENSITIVITY AND SPECIFICITY

(75%). This is because there were 24 participants whose falls status indicated they were recurrent fallers who also scored less than 20 on the POAM of the 32 who were recorded as recurrent fallers. The specificity in this example was $15/18 = 0.83$ (83%) because there were 15 participants who were not recurrent fallers who scored 20 or more on the POAM of the 18 participants who were not recurrent fallers.

Specificity and sensitivity should be balanced and at a level as high as possible because a screening test should ensure the highest percentage of true positives, and therefore the lowest percentage of false positives. However, specificity and sensitivity are inversely related, such that as one increases, the other decreases. These are participants who are test positive (having a score <20 on the POAM in the example shown in Figure 8.14), but are true negatives (in this example this equates to participants not having fallen recurrently). In the SPSS output shown in Figure 8.14 there are three false positives, that is those that did not fall recurrently (their true status) but their test performance showed they were at risk of recurrent falls (their test status). Likewise, it is necessary to minimise the number of false negatives. These are the participants who are test negative, but are true positives.

Two other quantities that are also often used in association with sensitivity and specificity are positive predictive value (PPV) and negative predictive value (NPV). Positive predictive value is the proportion (percentage) of participants who are test positive who are true positive. In the example shown in Figure 8.15 this is calculated using $24/27 = 0.89$ (89%). Negative predictive value is the proportion (percentage) of participants who are test negative who are true negative. Continuing

POAM with a cut off of 20 * Falls Status Crosstabulation

| | | | Falls Status | | Total |
			Not fallen recurrently	Fallen recurrently	
POAM with a cut off of 20	Not at risk of recurrent falling	Count % within POAM with a cut off of 20	15 65.2%	8 34.8%	23 100.0%
	At risk of recurrent falling	Count % within POAM with a cut off of 20	3 11.1%	24 88.9%	27 100.0%
Total		Count % within POAM with a cut off of 20	18 36.0%	32 64.0%	50 100.0%

Negative predictive value – the proportion (percentage) of those who are test negative who are true negative

Positive predictive value – the proportion (percentage) of those who are test positive who are true positive

FIGURE 8.15   CROSSTABULATION OF RECURRENT FALLS STATUS AND POAM SHOWING POSITIVE AND NEGATIVE PREDICTIVE VALUES

the example being used to illustrate this concept the negative predictive value is $15/23 = 0.65$ (65%). These percentages are calculated by SPSS by requesting row percentages if the true status is shown in the columns as shown in Figure 8.15.

Ninety-five percent confidence intervals can be calculated for all these statistics: sensitivity, specificity, positive predictive value and negative predictive value. However, as SPSS does not explicitly calculate sensitivity, specificity, positive and negative predictive values, it does not calculate the associated 95% confidence intervals routinely either, however, where possible these should be presented. Details on how to calculate these can be found in Bland (2000).

RECEIVER OPERATING CHARACTERISTIC (ROC) CURVES

Despite the POAM being treated as a categorical variable defined by a cut-off of less than 20 versus 20+ to indicate those who were and were not more likely to fall recurrently, the original POAM was actually a continuous variable. The cut-off did not come about by deciding that 20 was a 'nice' round number that would be easy to remember. It was brought about statistically by maximising both the sensitivity and specificity. Sensitivity and 1-specificity are plotted on a ROC curve so the relationship between these two quantities can be examined. A sensitivity of 1 and a specificity of 1 would show a vertical line up the left hand side of the plot (where 1-specificity = 0) area to a sensitivity of 1, then a horizontal line across the top of the plot to a 1-specificity of 1. This rarely happens; so on a ROC curve the point closest to the top left of the plot area will be the point at which the sensitivity and specificity are maximised.

The area under the curve is given in the output for ROC curves. It equals 1 when sensitivity and specificity equal 1 and it equals 0.5 when sensitivity and specificity equal 0. Therefore, the greater the area under the curve the better the test is at distinguishing between those with and without the disease or condition. If a number of tests are being considered to discover which is most efficient with regard to the 'gold standard' then a significance test to compare the areas under the curve can be carried out. However, this cannot be carried out in SPSS.

In SPSS, ROC curves are invoked by clicking on Analyze → ROC Curve ... to give the dialog box shown in Figure 8.16. On this dialog box, put the continuous variable in the Test Variable: box (in this example it is the continuous POAM score), and the dichotomous variable indicating the 'gold standard' in the State Variable: box (in this example it is the actual falls status). To accompany the State Variable: the value indicating when this is positive should be put in the Value of State Variable: box. In this example falls status is coded 1 if the participant is a recurrent faller (and 0 otherwise), so 1 is placed in the Value of State Variable: box. The only other information that is requested from this dialog box is Coordinate points of the ROC Curve. By requesting these, it can easily be seen where sensitivity and specificity are maximised, and thus where the cut-off should be.

Next click on the Options ... button to give the ROC Curve: Options dialog box shown in Figure 8.17. In this box, under the Test Direction, make sure the radio button relating to the correct direction of the test is selected. In the POAM example, a lower score indicates a lower level of balance. Therefore, in this context the radio button

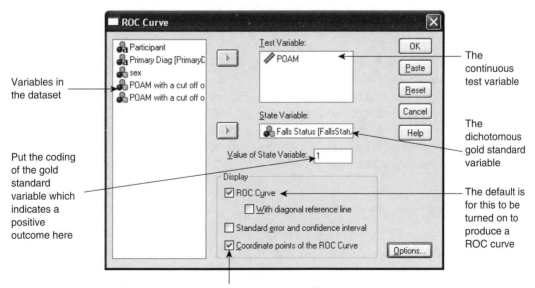

Variables in the dataset

The continuous test variable

The dichotomous gold standard variable

Put the coding of the gold standard variable which indicates a positive outcome here

The default is for this to be turned on to produce a ROC curve

Tick this box to give the sensitivity and 1-specificity at each point of the continuous variable

FIGURE 8.16   ROC CURVE DIALOG BOX

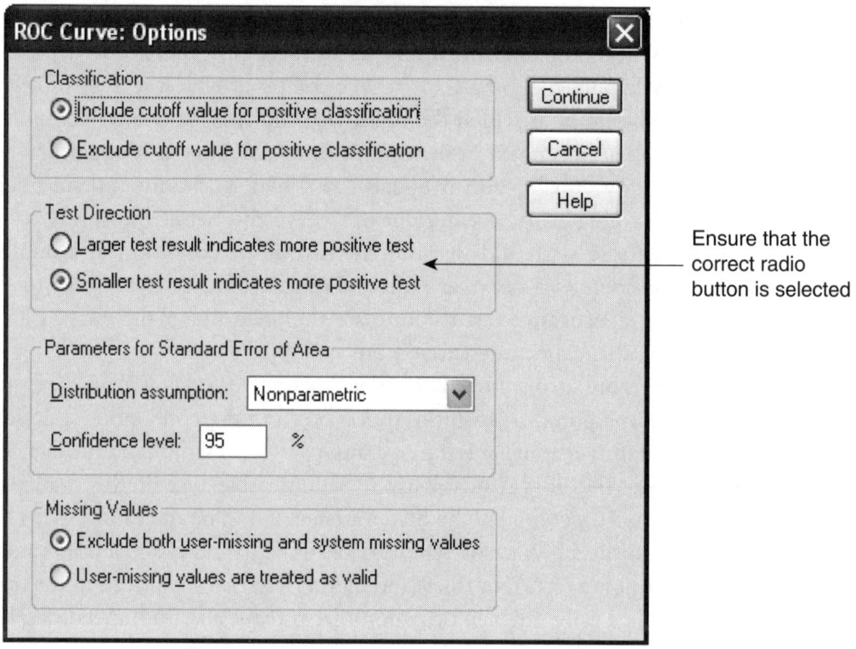

FIGURE 8.17   ROC CURVE: OPTIONS DIALOG BOX

indicating Smaller test result indicates more positive test should be selected. When this has been selected, click Continue to return to the ROC Curve dialog box (Figure 8.16) and then click OK to give the output shown in Figure 8.18.

Interpretation

From the Coordinates of the Curve table, the values of the sensitivities and 1–specificities are shown for each value of the POAM. It is shown with the rectangle that the POAM score that maximises the sensitivity and specificity is 19 or less (shown earlier in the chapter as <20 versus 20+), whereby the sensitivity is 0.75 (75%) and the specificity is $(1–0.167 = 0.833$ (83%)). This means that 75% of true positives are correctly identified by the test, and 83% of true negatives are correctly identified by the test. The area under the curve is 0.87.

SUMMARY

- Crosstabulations, Chi-square test, Fisher's exact test, sensitivity and specificity analysis and Cohen's Kappa are all invoked by going to the Crosstabs dialog box using Analyze → Descriptive Statistics → Crosstabs ... then selecting the appropriate options from that dialog box.
- For crosstabulation only, the only option needed is Row and/or Column percentages from the Cells ... dialog box.

ROC Curve

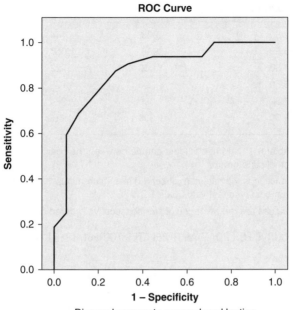

Diagonal segments are produced by ties

Area Under the Curve

Test Result Variable(s): POAM

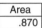

Area
.870

The test result variable(s): POAM has at least one tie between the positive actual state group and the negative actual state group. Statistics may be biased.

Coordinates of the Curve

Test Result Variable(s): POAM

Positive if Less Than or Equal to[a]	Sensitivity	1 – Specificity
6.00	.000	.000
7.50	.031	.000
8.50	.094	.000
9.50	.125	.000
11.00	.188	.000
12.50	.250	.056
13.50	.313	.056
14.50	.375	.056
15.50	.469	.056
16.50	.500	.056
17.50	.594	.056
18.50	.688	.111
19.50	.750	.167
20.50	.875	.278
21.50	.906	.333

(Continued)

FIGURE 8.18   (*Continued*)

22.50	.938	.444
23.50	.938	.667
24.50	1.000	.722
25.50	1.000	.778
27.00	1.000	.944
29.00	1.000	1.000

The test result variable(s): POAM has at least one tie between the positive actual state group and the negative actual state group.

[a] The smallest cutoff value is the minimum observed test value minus 1, and the largest cutoff value is the maximum observed test value plus 1.

All the other cutoff values are the averages of two consecutive ordered observed test values.

FIGURE 8.18   ROC CURVE FOR POAM AS IT RELATES TO RECURRENT FALLS

- For the chi-square test, the Chi-Square box should be ticked in the Statistics ... dialog box.
- For Fisher's exact test, the Chi-Square box should be ticked in the Statistics ... dialog box and the Exact radio button should be selected in the Exact dialog box.
- Cohen's Kappa is requested by ticking the Kappa box from the Statistics ... button on the Crosstabs dialog box.
- ROC curves are invoked from Analyze → ROC Curves....

EXERCISES

1   In the paper by De Tychey et al. (2008), the authors state that one of the null hypotheses of the study was 'PND will not be higher in frequency for French women if the baby is female' (PND is post natal depression). Data produced took the form of a three (level of PND) by two (child gender) crosstabulation. How could the null hypothesis be altered to test all possible situations that might arise from the data?

2   What would the alternative hypothesis to go with the altered null hypothesis suggested in Question 1 be?

Open smoking.sav.

3   Construct a crosstabulation using SPSS for smoking status and perceived length of smokers' breaks. How many current smokers think smokers' breaks are longer than non-smokers' breaks?

4   Carry out an appropriate significance test on these two variables. Which statistical test did you use?

5 Was there a statistically significant relationship between smoking status and perceived length of smokers' breaks?

Table 8.2 shows the cut off from the measures listed that best predict a Bayley MDI<70 (Bayley, 1993) at age two in children born extremely preterm. An MDI<70 indicates neurological developmental delay. Linguistic skills comprise vocabulary and sentence complexity. Parent report composite comprises non-verbal cognition, vocabulary and sentence complexity (Johnson et al., 2004).

TABLE 8.2 ROC CURVE DETERMINED PARENT REPORT CUT-OFF SCORES FOR PREDICTION OF MDI SCORE OF LESS THAN 70

Measure	Cut off	Sensitivity (95% CI)	Specificity (95% CI)
Vocabulary	18	0.81 (0.41, 0.89)	0.71 (0.67, 0.91)
Sentence complexity	7	0.81 (0.54, 0.96)	0.67 (0.52, 0.80)
Linguistic skills	30	0.81 (0.54, 0.96)	0.77 (0.63, 0.88)
Parent report composite	49	0.81 (0.54, 0.96)	0.81 (0.67, 0.91)

ROC – receiver operating characteristic; MDI – Mental Development Index

6 What does sensitivity indicate?
7 What is the advantage of selecting the parent report composite as the means of predicting children who may have an MDI score <70?

Table 8.3 is a crosstabulation of age at menarche recorded at two time points. This was established during a medical examination at age 14–15 and through a postal questionnaire at age 48 (Cooper et al., 2006).

TABLE 8.3 CROSSTABULATION OF CATEGORIES OF AGE AT MENARCHE DERIVED FROM AGES OF MENARCHE ASCERTAINED DURING ADOLESCENCE AND IN MIDDLE AGE IN THE MEDICAL RESEARCH COUNCIL NATIONAL SURVEY OF HEALTH AND DEVELOPMENT COHORT (N = 1050)

		Age at menarche (years) recorded at age 14–15 years			
		≤11	12–13	≥14	Total
Age at menarche (years) recorded at age 48 years	≤11	122 (71)	144 (22)	2 (1)	268
	12–13	45 (26)	386 (59)	44 (20)	475
	≥4	4 (2)	126 (19)	177 (79)	307
	Total	171	656	223	1050

Values are n (%)

8 How many women agreed on their grouping of age at menarche?
9 Kappa for this Table was 0.43. What does this indicate about agreement between the two time points?
10 Looking at the data shown in Table 8.3, if you were doing a study of middle aged women, would it be worthwhile asking the women about their age at menarche?

9
COMPARING MEANS

INTRODUCTION

Once continuous data have been explored using summary statistics as shown in Chapter 5, it may be appropriate to discover whether means are significantly different between groups. This chapter will use parametric tests; which have assumptions about the data that have to be satisfied before the test can be used with a given variable. Statistical tests for continuous data which do not have such assumptions are explored in Chapter 10.

Where there are two groups the independent samples t-test should be used. Where there are more than two groups the most appropriate statistical test is the one-way analysis of variance (ANOVA). Sometimes the same measurement is taken on the same participants at two or more time points, for example lung function before and after exercise, blood pressure before and after an intervention or the same outcome measure being completed at a number of time points. The paired t-test can be used to determine whether there is a difference in means between two time points, or where cases and controls are matched. Where there are more than two time points, the repeated measures ANOVA should be used.

This chapter will use data from the student obesity data, whereby students collected data on opinions of causes and effects of obesity as well as demographic information and height and weight. It will also use data from the United Kingdom Oscillation Study (UKOS) (Johnson et al., 2002) to illustrate comparisons of means at a number of time points.

THE AIMS OF THIS CHAPTER ARE:

- To understand when it is appropriate to use a given test to compare means.
- To learn how to compare means between two groups using SPSS.
- To learn how to compare means between more than two groups.
- To learn how to compare means where data are paired.
- To interpret results gained from analysis using SPSS.

INDEPENDENT SAMPLES T-TEST

The independent samples t-test (sometime also called the two samples t-test or unpaired t-test) is used to discover whether there are statistically significant differences in means between two groups. This means that a continuous variable and a dichotomous variable are required in order to carry out the independent samples t-test. This test can be used to answer such questions as 'Is there a difference in mean height between boys and girls of a given age?' or 'Is there a difference in mean blood pressure between white and non-white people?' In these examples height and blood pressure are the continuous variables; gender and ethnicity are the dichotomous variables. The independent samples t-test has two assumptions that should be satisfied to make the test valid. The first is that the data are Normally distributed; the other being that the variances (related to the standard deviation) of the two groups are equal. When using real data, it is unlikely that the distributions will follow the standard Normal distribution exactly, nor that the variances will be exactly the same; but data should be close to Normally distributed with similar variances. In addition participants should be independent of one another (in its simplest form, all data should be from different participants).

Transformation

If the continuous variable is not Normally distributed (check using a histogram), it may be possible to transform the variable to yield a variable which is closer to Normal which can be used for analysis using the independent samples t-test. Transformations using natural logarithms or by taking the square root of the data may be possible. If this is not possible, a non-parametric test could be used. This is explained further in Chapter 10.

Back to the independent samples t-test

At the outset the null and alternative hypotheses for the independent samples t-test have to be set up. These take the general form:

H$_0$: There is no mean difference in the continuous variable between the dichotomous variable's categories.

H$_1$: There is a mean difference in the continuous variable between the dichotomous variable's categories.

The data used in this example are from the student obesity dataset. Within the questionnaire, participants were asked to give their weight. This analysis will compare mean weights between males and females.

Before the independent samples t-test can be carried out, the assumption that the continuous variable in question is Normally distributed by group should be

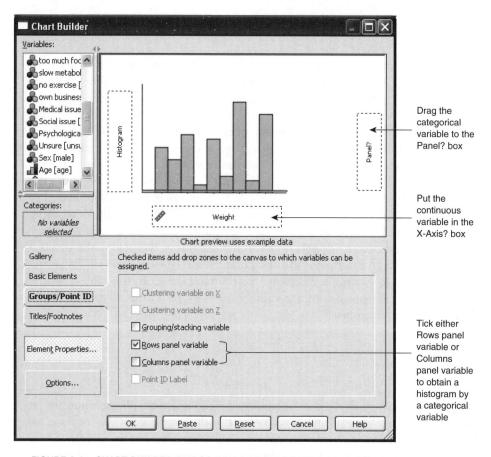

FIGURE 9.1   CHART BUILDER DIALOG BOX SHOWING PANELLED HISTOGRAM

checked. To do this, create a histogram by the two groups. The construction of simple histograms using SPSS is shown in Chapter 5. To make the histogram show data by a categorical variable, click the Groups/Point ID tab on the Chart Builder dialog box. On that tab either tick Rows panel variable (to produce graphs like those in Figure 9.2) or Columns panel variable (to produce the graphs side by side). Drag the grouping variable (sex in this example) to the Panel? box so that the dialog box looks like that shown in Figure 9.1 to give the histograms shown in Figure 9.2.

The specific null and alternative hypotheses to be tested are:

H_0: There is no mean difference in weight between males and females.
H_1: There is a mean difference in weight between males and females.

To obtain an independent samples t-test using SPSS, click on Analyze → Compare Means → Independent-Samples T Test … . This will give the dialog box shown in Figure 9.3. Put the continuous variable (weight in this example) in the Test Variable(s): box and the dichotomous variable (gender) in the Grouping Variable box. When a variable has been placed in the Grouping Variable: box, it is necessary to click the Define Groups… button to proceed. This will give the dialog box shown

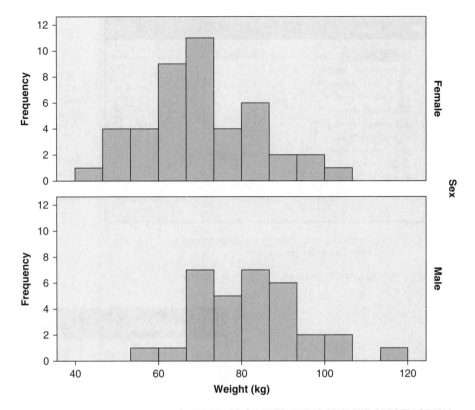

FIGURE 9.2   HISTOGRAM OF WEIGHT OF PARTICIPANTS IN THE STUDENT OBESITY STUDY BY GENDER

in Figure 9.4: In the Group 1: and Group 2: boxes, the coding for the dichotomous variable should be declared. This can be checked using Variable View. For example, in this dataset, females were coded 0 and males were coded 1, so 0 was placed in the box next to Group 1: and 1 in the box next to Group 2:. When the groups have been defined, click on Continue to return to the Independent-Samples T Test dialog box (Figure 9.3), followed by OK to obtain the output (Figure 9.5).

Interpretation

Figure 9.2 shows that weight is Normally distributed for both genders. As would be expected, it can be seen that the minimum weight is lower in females than males whilst the reverse is true for the maximum. Using Figure 9.5, it can be seen that the mean weight for females is 70kg (SD 13kg) and 82kg (SD 12kg) for males. The mean difference in weight (females minus males) is −12.3kg (95% CI −18.3kg, −6.4kg). This means we are 95% certain that the true population mean difference could be as much as 18.3kg (females could be on average 18.3kg lighter than males in the population) or as little as 6.4kg (females could be on average 6.4kg lighter than males in the population). This is a significant difference in means ($p < 0.001$).

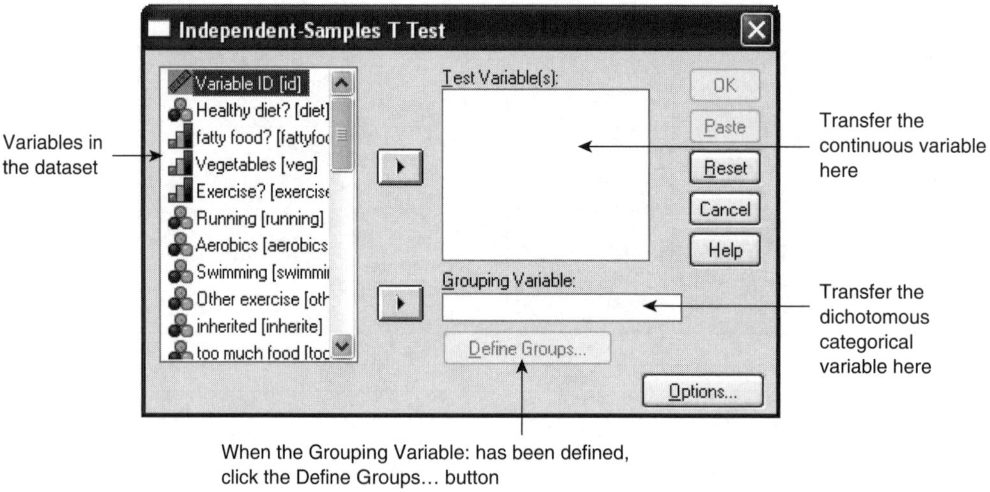

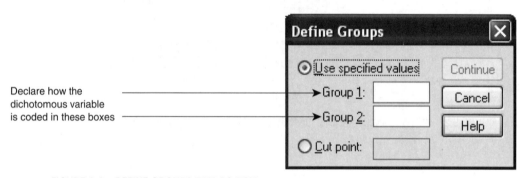

FIGURE 9.3   INDEPENDENT-SAMPLES T TEST DIALOG BOX

FIGURE 9.4   DEFINE GROUPS DIALOG BOX

Equal variances

The other assumption of the independent samples t-test is that the variances are equal. To check this, in the independent samples t-test output in SPSS, look at the standard deviations of the two groups (Figure 9.5, Group Statistics). In the example shown in Figure 9.5 the standard deviations are 13.1 and 12.4 for females and males respectively, which, although are not the same, are sufficiently close for the assumption of equal variances to hold.

If the standard deviation is larger in the group with the larger mean, this may be indicative of the data being skew, and transformation may be necessary (Peacock and Kerry, 2007). SPSS also provides Levene's Test for Equality of Variance in the Independent Samples Test output. However, this is of limited use since the test may not indicate important differences as being significant when the dataset is small. Conversely, a small difference in the variance that would not affect the modelling is sometimes shown to be significant when the dataset is larger (Peacock and Kerry, 2007); therefore, it is better to assess variance by eye using the summary statistics. A p-value <0.05 with Levene's Test for Equality of Variance indicates that the variances

Group Statistics

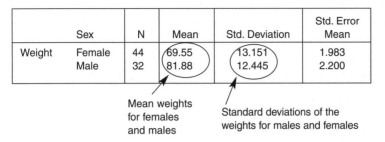

	Sex	N	Mean	Std. Deviation	Std. Error Mean
Weight	Female	44	69.55	13.151	1.983
	Male	32	81.88	12.445	2.200

Mean weights for females and males

Standard deviations of the weights for males and females

Independent Samples Text

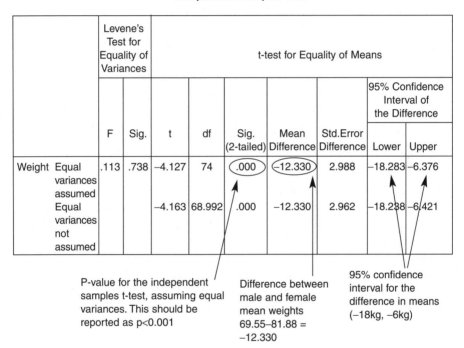

		Levene's Test for Equality of Variances		t-test for Equality of Means					95% Confidence Interval of the Difference	
		F	Sig.	t	df	Sig. (2-tailed)	Mean Difference	Std.Error Difference	Lower	Upper
Weight	Equal variances assumed	.113	.738	−4.127	74	.000	−12.330	2.988	−18.283	−6.376
	Equal variances not assumed			−4.163	68.992	.000	−12.330	2.962	−18.238	−6.421

P-value for the independent samples t-test, assuming equal variances. This should be reported as p<0.001

Difference between male and female mean weights
69.55−81.88 = −12.330

95% confidence interval for the difference in means (−18kg, −6kg)

FIGURE 9.5   INDEPENDENT SAMPLES T-TEST, BIRTHWEIGHT AND SEX.

are not equal. If the variances are not equal, then there is a modified independent samples t–test, with statistics given on the row Equal variances not assumed (Figure 9.5). SPSS calculates t–tests assuming and not assuming equal variances whenever an independent samples t–test is requested, and the user should be careful to use the appropriate output.

One-way Analysis of Variance (ANOVA)

One-way ANOVA is a natural extension of the independent samples t–test. It is used to compare means between more than two groups. It is worth noting that a series of independent samples t-tests should not be used when there are more than two groups because there would be a large number of pairwise tests that could be undertaken (especially when there are a large number of groups), and with increasing numbers of tests undertaken, the probability of one difference in means being sufficiently large to be significant increases.

The general null and alternative hypotheses for the one-way ANOVA are:

H_0: There is no mean difference in the continuous variable between the categorical variable's categories.

H_1: There is a mean difference in the continuous variable between the categorical variable's categories.

As with the independent samples t-test the one-way ANOVA has two assumptions. The first being that the data are Normally distributed within groups. This can be checked using histograms as for the independent samples t-test. The other assumption is that the variances are equal. SPSS does not give a formal test to explore this, but descriptive statistics by group can be scrutinised and a judgement made on that basis.

The one-way ANOVA will be explained using the same student obesity dataset, this time using age in three categories.

The specific hypotheses to be tested in the following example are:

H_0: There is no difference in mean weight between age groups.

H_1: There is a difference in mean weight between age groups.

To invoke the one way ANOVA, click on Analyze → Compare Means → One-Way ANOVA....This will give the dialog box shown in Figure 9.6. In this dialog box, move the continuous variable (weight in this example) to the Dependent List: box and the categorical variable with three or more categories (age group in this example) to the Factor: box.Then click the Options… button to get the dialog box shown in Figure 9.7. From this dialog box tick Descriptive to request descriptive statistics related to the variables selected in the One-Way ANOVA dialog box (Figure 9.6), then click Continue to return to the One-Way ANOVA dialog box (Figure 9.6). Finally click OK to obtain the output (Figure 9.8).

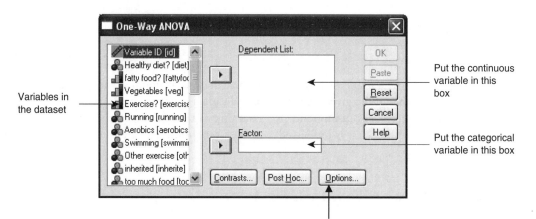

FIGURE 9.6 ONE-WAY ANOVA DIALOG BOX

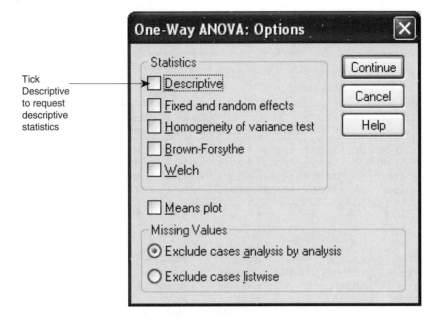

Tick
Descriptive
to request
descriptive
statistics

FIGURE 9.7   ONE-WAY ANOVA: OPTIONS DIALOG BOX

Interpretation

Figure 9.8 shows the mean weight of participants in kg by age group (11 to 30 years, 31 to 40 years and 41+ years). It shows that the mean weight ranges from 74.0kg (SD 15.6kg) for the 11 to 30 year old age group to 75.6kg (SD 12.3) for the 31 to 40 year old age group. There is not a statistically significant difference in mean weight between the three age groups (p=0.897). This indicates a significant difference in mean weight has not been shown and the null hypothesis can be accepted.

PAIRED T-TEST

The paired t-test is used when the same measurement is taken before and after an intervention (or just at different time points) on the same participants; for example lung function test taken before and after exercise. It can also be utilised when a continuous outcome is measured on the same participants using two different pieces of equipment to determine whether the mean outcome between the two pieces of equipment differs significantly. For example, measuring blood pressure using two makes of sphagmometers to determine whether their measurements are equivalent. Finally, the paired t-test can also be used to compare means of a continuous outcome in matched cases and controls.

As data are paired, it implies that there has to be the same number of observations at both time points, and that the data at the two time points form a pair by the participant being measured twice (or the case and control both providing data). If data are missing at one time point but not the other, then that participant is not used in the analysis. There are two assumptions of the paired t-test that have to be met: the first is that the differences between the two values (for example, blood pressure at two

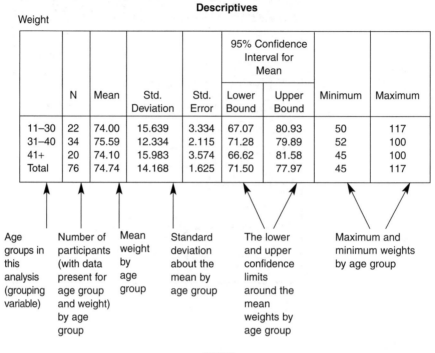

Descriptives

Weight

	N	Mean	Std. Deviation	Std. Error	95% Confidence Interval for Mean		Minimum	Maximum
					Lower Bound	Upper Bound		
11–30	22	74.00	15.639	3.334	67.07	80.93	50	117
31–40	34	75.59	12.334	2.115	71.28	79.89	52	100
41+	20	74.10	15.983	3.574	66.62	81.58	45	100
Total	76	74.74	14.168	1.625	71.50	77.97	45	117

Age groups in this analysis (grouping variable) | Number of participants (with data present for age group and weight) by age group | Mean weight by age group | Standard deviation about the mean by age group | The lower and upper confidence limits around the mean weights by age group | Maximum and minimum weights by age group

ANOVA

Weight

	Sum of Squares	df	Mean Square	F	Sig.	
Between Groups	44.702	2	22.351	.109	.897	p-value for the one-way ANOVA
Within Groups	15010.035	73	205.617			
Total	15054.737	75				

FIGURE 9.8   WEIGHT BY AGE GROUP DESCRIPTIVE STATISTICS AND ONE-WAY ANOVA

time points) are Normally distributed, although the actual values at the two time points do not have to be Normally distributed; the other assumption is that the differences are independent of one another. This means that each pair of observations should come from a different participant.

The general null and alternative hypotheses for the paired t-test are:

H_0: There is no difference in means between the two time points/between cases and controls.
H_1: There is a difference in means between the two time points/between cases and controls.

Before carrying out the paired t-test, the assumption that the changes or differences between the two variables are Normally distributed should be tested. To do this using SPSS, compute a new variable giving the difference between the two variables using Transform → Compute Variable… then following the procedure described in Chapter 2.

When the difference variable has been constructed, check its distribution using a histogram (Chapter 5). If the difference variable is Normally distributed, the paired t-test can be used. If the difference variable is skewed, then the paired t-test cannot be used unless both the paired variables are transformed. The differences should then be recalculated to determine whether they are Normally distributed. Alternative tests that can be used when the differences are not Normally distributed are illustrated in Chapter 10.

The data used in this example are from UKOS. The specific variables to be used are blood pressure at 2 and 12 hours after birth, making the paired t-test appropriate because the same variable is being tested on the same participants at two time points. These give the following specific null and alternative hypotheses:

H_0: There is no difference in mean blood pressure between 2 hours and 12 hours of age.
H_1: There is a difference in mean blood pressure between 2 hours and 12 hours of age.

The histogram of the differences of the data used in this example is shown in Figure 9.9. The histogram shows that the mean difference between blood pressure at 2 hours and blood pressure at 12 hours is 3.8mmHg (SD 9.1mmHg). The histogram does not show a perfectly Normal distribution, but this is expected in real data and it is close enough to be able to use the paired t-test. A difference of 0 would indicate that blood pressure at 2 hours was the same as blood pressure at 12 hours. There were a few extreme differences, for example, the differences of greater than 30mmHg indicate that blood pressure at 2 hours was more than 30mmHg greater than blood pressure at 12 hours.

The paired t-test can be selected using Analyze → Compare Means → Paired-Samples t-test… to give a dialog box as in Figure 9.10. From the list of variables in the dataset, variables have to be selected in pairs. Both variables will appear in the Current Selections section of the Paired Samples T Test dialog box (Figure 9.10) until they are moved to the Paired Variables: box by clicking the arrow (▶). When at least one pair of variables has been moved to the Paired Variables: box, click OK to give the output shown in Figure 9.11.

Interpretation

Data from 75 participants were analysed. The mean blood pressure at 2 hours was 34mmHg (Figure 9.11), whilst the mean blood pressure at 12 hours was 31mmHg (95% confidence interval for the difference 1.7mmHg, 5.9mmHg). This was statistically significant $p = 0.001$, meaning that a significant difference in mean blood pressure between 2 hours and 12 hours has been shown (consistent with the alternative hypothesis).

Notice this interpretation gives the 95% confidence interval for the difference to one decimal place (fewer decimal places than in Figure 9.11). There is no need to report such information to more than one decimal place; in doing so spurious precision will be introduced especially given that blood pressure is only measured to the nearest mmHg.

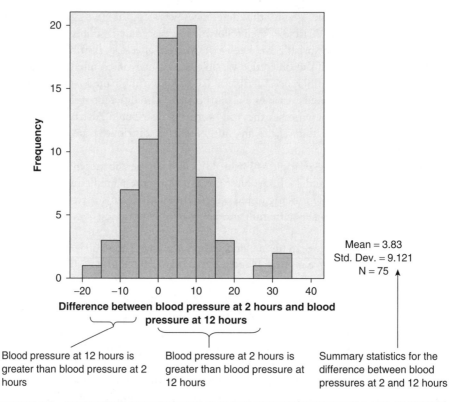

Mean = 3.83
Std. Dev. = 9.121
N = 75

Difference between blood pressure at 2 hours and blood pressure at 12 hours

Blood pressure at 12 hours is greater than blood pressure at 2 hours

Blood pressure at 2 hours is greater than blood pressure at 12 hours

Summary statistics for the difference between blood pressures at 2 and 12 hours

FIGURE 9.9   HISTOGRAM OF DIFFERENCE IN BLOOD PRESSURE BETWEEN 2 AND 12 HOURS FOLLOWING BIRTH IN INFANTS BORN EXTREMELY PRETERM

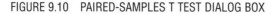

Variables in the dataset

Selected variables appear in this box before the

▶ button is pressed

Selected variables move to this box when the arrow button is pressed

FIGURE 9.10   PAIRED-SAMPLES T TEST DIALOG BOX

REPEATED MEASURES ANOVA

Where measurements are taken on participants at more than two time points, it is statistically correct to test the overall difference in continuous outcome between time points, and not to test all possible pairwise differences because of the problems

Paired Samples Statistics

		Mean	N	Std. Deviation	Std. Error Mean	
Pair 1	Blood pressure at 2 hours	34.45	75	7.664	.885	Summary statistics for the two variables analysed
	Blood pressure at 12 hours	30.63	75	6.501	.751	

Paired Samples Correlations

		N	Correlation	Sig.
Pair 1	Blood pressure at 2 hours & Blood pressure at 12 hours	75	.179	.125

Correlation coefficient and p-value for the two variables analysed. See Chapter 11 for more details on correlation

Paired Samples Test

		Paired Differences							
					95% Confidence Interval of the Difference				
		Mean	Std. Deviation	Std. Error Mean	Lower	Upper	t	df	Sig. (2-tailed)
Pair 1	Blood pressure at 2 hours – Blood pressure at 12 hours	3.827	9.121	1.053	1.728	5.925	3.633	74	.001

Difference between mean blood pressure at 2 hours and mean blood pressure at 12 hours. (34.45–30.63)

95% confidence interval for the difference between means

P-value for the paired t-test

FIGURE 9.11   PAIRED T-TEST, BLOOD PRESSURE AT 2 AND 12 HOURS AFTER BIRTH

associated with multiple testing. This can be done using the repeated measures ANOVA. This description will be limited to the simplest situation where the means of the outcome variables are being compared between time points; that is, no other variables are being taken into account in analysis.

As with other parametric tests explained in this chapter there are a number of assumptions that must be satisfied for the repeated measures ANOVA to be valid. The first involves normality; with data within each time point being Normally distributed. As shown previously this can be examined using histograms. Variances within data from each time point are assumed to be equal. Finally, participants should be independent of one another. Additionally, in common with the paired t-test, only participants that have data present at all time points are included in the analysis.

As with the paired t-test example, the data for this example come from UKOS, specifically the same variables, namely blood pressure after birth are used. This time blood measurements at three time points are used (2 hours, 12 hours and 24 hours following birth). Under normal circumstances if data are available for more than two time points the repeated measure would be the statistical method of choice to avoid multiple testing resulting from carrying out a large number of pairwise analyses.

To invoke a one-way repeated measures ANOVA in SPSS click on Analyze → General Linear Model → Repeated Measures....This will give the Repeated Measures Define Factor(s) dialog box (Figure 9.12). In this dialog box the Within Subject Factor Name: box has to be filled. Using the data for this example, the repeated factor is time so this name can be used in this box (although the actual name is arbitrary and could be left at the default of factor1 as long as this is not going to cause confusion when interpreting the output). The Number of Levels: box also has to be filled. This equates to the number of repeats in the data; so with the example being used to illustrate this test, this would be three. Once both of these boxes have been filled the Define button will become functional; click it to get the Repeated Measures dialog box shown in Figure 9.13. Within this dialog box the variables that represent the time points should be transferred from the variable list to the Within Subjects Variables (time): box. In the context of the ongoing example, these are the three variables giving the blood pressure measurements at the three time points. As no other variables are being included in the analysis, neither of the other boxes in Figure 9.13 needs to be filled.

Next click on the Options... button on the Repeated Measures dialog box (Figure 9.13) to give the Repeated Measures: Options dialog box (Figure 9.14). From the Factor(s) and Factor Interactions: box move the factor created in Figure 9.12 (time in this example) to the Display Means for: box. OVERALL is also displayed in the

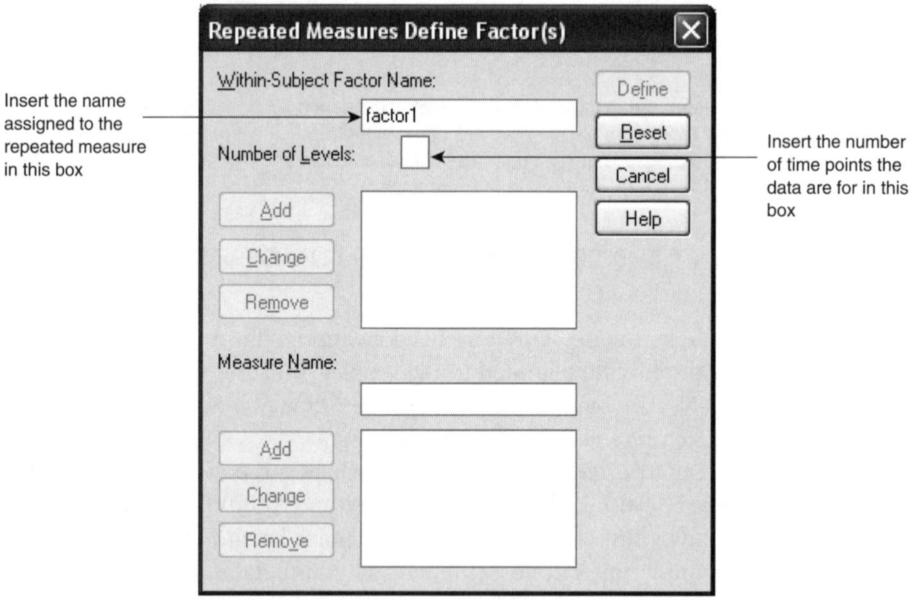

FIGURE 9.12   REPEATED MEASURES DEFINE FACTOR(S) DIALOG BOX

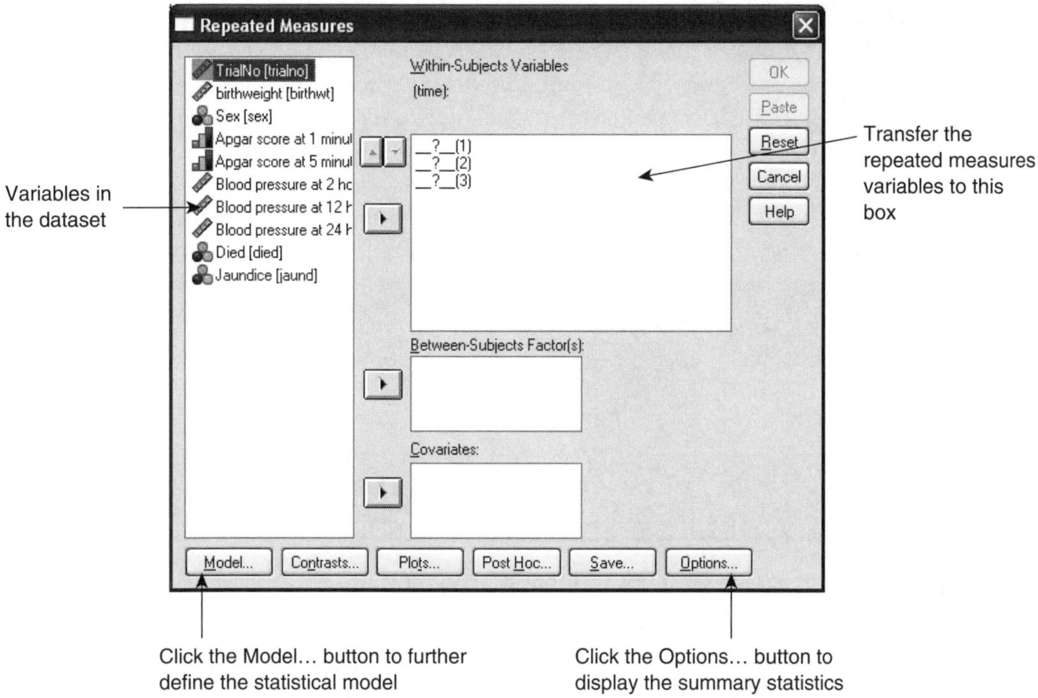

Variables in the dataset

Transfer the repeated measures variables to this box

Click the Model... button to further define the statistical model

Click the Options... button to display the summary statistics

FIGURE 9.13   REPEATED MEASURES DIALOG BOX

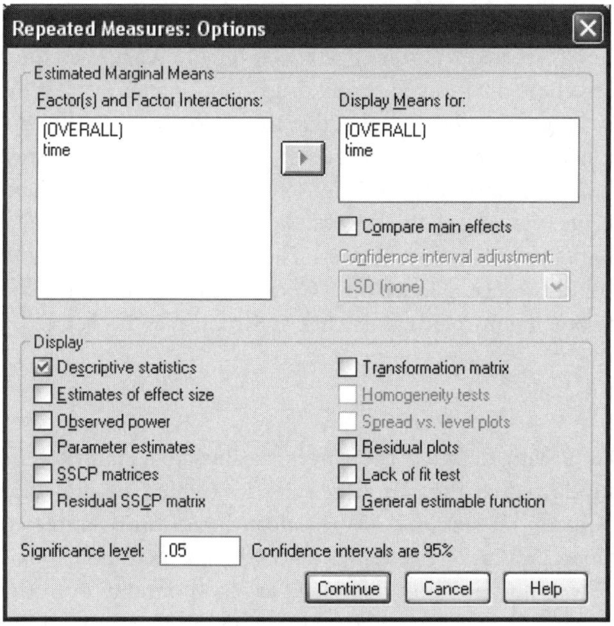

FIGURE 9.14   REPEATED MEASURES: OPTIONS DIALOG BOX

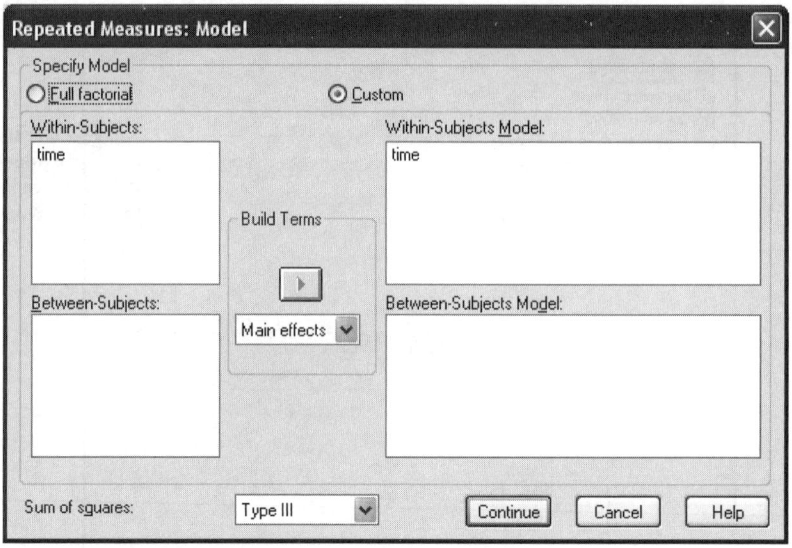

FIGURE 9.15   REPEATED MEASURES: MODEL DIALOG BOX

Factor(s) and Factor Interactions: box. If this is also transferred to the Display Means for: box, statistics for the three factors (that is blood pressure at 2 hours, 12 hours and 24 hours), combined will be shown. It is likely that this will have limited value because it is far more useful and informative to give summary statistics of the outcome (blood pressure) separately at the three time points. Then tick Descriptive statistics under Display. When all options have been specified, click the Continue button to return to the Repeated Measures dialog box.

Then, from the Repeated Measures dialog box (Figure 9.13), click the on Model button to give the Repeated Measures: model dialog box (Figure 9.15). Whilst there are no covariates in the model, it is not essential that this dialog box is changed as there is only one model that could be produced, however it is good practice to get used to setting the appropriate options. The first thing to do is to select the Custom radio button, then under Build Terms change the drop down box that contains Interaction as the default to Main effects (giving a model without interactions). Then transfer time from the Within-Subjects box to the Within-Subjects Model box. Click Continue to return to the Repeated Measures dialog box (Figure 9.13), then click OK to invoke the output (Figure 9.16).

Interpretation

Figure 9.16 starts with defining the three variables that constitute the three time points. This is followed by the summary statistics (which are also shown at the end of the output). It can be seen that 72 participants had data available at all three time points. Mean blood pressures ranged from 30.6 (SD 6.5) at 12 hours to 35.0 (SD 6.5) at 24 hours. There was no significant difference in blood pressure over time (p = 0.494). The p-value is circled in Figure 9.16. Note this result is very different from the result of the paired t-test shown earlier in this chapter. This is because the mean blood pressures at 2 hours and 24 hours were very close to one another.

Within-Subjects Factors

Measure: MEASURE_1

time	Dependent Variable
1	bp2
2	bp12
3	bp24

Descriptive Statistics

	Mean	Std. Deviation	N
Blood pressure at 2 hours	34.29	7.583	72
Blood pressure at 12 hours	30.63	6.547	72
Blood pressure at 24 hours	35.00	6.502	72

Multivariate Tests[b]

Effect		Value	F	Hypothesis df	Error df	Sig.
time	Pillai's Trace	.264	12.537[a]	2.000	70.000	.000
	Wilks' Lambda	.736	12.537[a]	2.000	70.000	.000
	Hotelling's Trace	.358	12.537[a]	2.000	70.000	.000
	Roy's Largest Root	.358	12.537[a]	2.000	70.000	.000

a. Exact statistic
b. Design: Intercept
Within Subjects Design: time

Mauchly's Test of Sphericity[b]

Measure: MEASURE_1

Within Subjects Effect	Mauchly's W	Approx. Chi-Square	df	Sig.	Epsilon[a]		
					Greenhouse-Geisser	Huynh-Feldt	Lower-bound
time	.952	3.421	2	.181	.954	.980	.500

Tests the null hypothesis that the error covariance matrix of the orthonormalized transformed dependent variables is proportional to an identity matrix.
a. May be used to adjust the degrees of freedom for the averaged tests of significance. Corrected tests are displayed in the Tests of Within-Subjects Effects table.
b. Design: Intercept
Within Subjects Design: time

(Continued)

FIGURE 9.16 (*Continued*)

Tests of Within-Subjects Effects

Measure: MEASURE_1

Source		Type III Sum of Squares	df	Mean Square	F	Sig.
time	Sphericity Assumed	794.083	2	397.042	10.901	.000
	Greenhouse-Geisser	794.083	1.909	415.980	10.901	.000
	Huynh-Feldt	794.083	1.960	405.068	10.901	.000
	Lower-bound	794.083	1.000	794.083	10.901	.002
Error(time)	Sphericity Assumed	5171.917	142	36.422		
	Greenhouse-Geisser	5171.917	135.535	38.159		
	Huynh-Feldt	5171.917	139.186	37.158		
	Lower-bound	5171.917	71.000	72.844		

Tests of Within-Subjects Contrasts

Measure: MEASURE_1

Source	time	Type III Sum of Squares	df	Mean Square	F	Sig.
time	Linear	18.063	1	18.063	.472	.494
	Quadratic	776.021	1	776.021	22.420	.000
Error(time)	Linear	2714.438	71	38.232		
	Quadratic	2457.479	71	34.612		

Tests of Between-Subjects Effects

Measure: MEASURE_1

Transformed Variable: Average

Source	Type III Sum of Squares	df	Mean Square	F	Sig.
Intercept	239600.167	1	239600.167	3432.644	.000
Error	4955.833	71	69.800		

1. Grand Mean

Measure: MEASURE_1

Mean	Std. Error	95% Confidence Interval	
		Lower Bound	Upper Bound
33.306	.568	32.172	34.439

2. Time

Measure: MEASURE_1

time	Mean	Std. Error	95% Confidence Interval	
			Lower Bound	Upper Bound
1	34.292	.894	32.510	36.074
2	30.625	.772	29.087	32.163
3	35.000	.766	33.472	36.528

FIGURE 9.16 REPEATED MEASURE ANOVA OUTPUT

SUMMARY

- The independent samples t-test is used to compare the means of two groups. It can be invoked using Analyze → Compare Means → Independent-Samples T Test... .
- The one-way analysis of variance is used to compare the means of more than two groups. It can be obtained using Analyze → Compare Means → One-Way ANOVA... .
- The paired t-test is used to analyse data from the same participants at two time points. The dialog box to undertake this method can be invoked using Analyze → Compare Means → Paired-Samples T Test... .
- The repeated measures ANOVA is the natural extension of the paired t-test. It is invoked in SPSS by clicking Analyze → General Linear Model → Repeated Measures... .

EXERCISES

Mean scores were higher in pregnancy than postnatally, with a peak at 32 weeks of pregnancy of 6.72 (SD 4.94) and a lowest value at 8 months postpartum (5.25 (4.61)). The mean change in depression score from that at 18 weeks of pregnancy was −0.097 (95% confidence interval −0.18 to −0.01, P = 0.025) at 32 weeks of pregnancy, 0.78 (0.69 to 0.88, P < 0.001) at 8 weeks postpartum, and 1.37 (1.27 to 1.46, P < 0.001) at 8 months postpartum. Mean change in score was 0.88 (0.79 to 0.97, P < 0.001) between 32 weeks of pregnancy and 8 weeks postpartum, 1.46 (1.37 to 1.56, P < 0.001) between 32 weeks of pregnancy and 8 months postpartum, and −0.58 (−0.50 to −0.67, P < 0.001) between 8 weeks and 8 months postpartum. (Evans et al., 2001: 258)

1 What statistical test was used to analyse the data described?
2 From the results given, what would you conclude about depression status in these women?
3 How could the analysis strategy of these data have been improved?

Open obesity.sav.

4 Do a comparison of mean weight between those who do and do not take any exercise. What is the mean (SD) weight for those who do and do not take any exercise? Is there a significant difference in weight between those who do and do not take any exercise?
5 Can a causal relationship between mean weight and exercise status be implied from the results shown in Question 4?

10
NON-PARAMETRIC TESTS

INTRODUCTION

Sometimes it is not possible to use the statistical tests described in Chapter 9 because the data violate the assumptions of those tests. For example, the data may be skewed and it is not possible to transform it. However, such data also need to be analysed because their results can make a valuable contribution to knowledge. For this situation an alternative set of statistical tests called non-parametric tests exist, they do not have any underlying assumptions.

This chapter will continue by describing a number of non-parametric tests one by one, including the circumstances in which they are used and examples of how to carry out the tests in SPSS.

This chapter will be illustrated using a small dataset of participants who were hospitalised as a result of stroke (n = 25) (Stein et al., 2009). They completed a number of outcome measures at admission, discharge and five weeks post discharge. Demographic data and information on their neglect (ignoring one half of the body or field of vision (Stroke Association, 2008)) status and discharge destination also comprised part of the dataset and will be used in the examples in this chapter.

THE AIMS OF THIS CHAPTER ARE:

- To learn when it is appropriate to use non-parametric tests, and which tests should be used in a given situation.
- To learn how to carry out non-parametric tests using SPSS.

PRELIMINARIES TO THIS CHAPTER

Many non-parametric tests use ranking. This involves putting the data in order of magnitude as was done to obtain the median in Chapter 5. The methods of calculating the test statistic for the individual tests in this chapter are beyond the scope of this book, but medians (and interquartile ranges or ranges) are usually presented with p-values resulting from non-parametric tests.

MANN-WHITNEY U TEST

This test is the non-parametric equivalent of the independent samples t-test. Therefore this test examines relationships between a continuous or ordered variable and a dichotomous variable. The only proviso for this test to be valid is that the data are ordinal (ordered, but the differences between data points do not have to have meaning). The Mann–Whitney U test does not provide any information on the central tendency like the tests in Chapter 9 do, such statistics have to be calculated using Descriptive Statistics in SPSS; with the median (interquartile range or range) being the most appropriate. The Mann–Whitney U test provides a p-value only.

As with other significance tests, null and alternative hypotheses have to be set up of the general form:

H_0: There is no tendency for members of one population to exceed members of the other in either direction in terms of the outcome in question.

H_1: There is a tendency for members of one population to exceed members of the other in either direction in terms of the outcome in question.

This example will determine whether there is a difference in scores at discharge on the Barthel Index between those who were discharged home and those who were discharged to an institution (Mahoney and Barthel, 1965). The Barthel Index measures activities of daily living and mobility on a scale which ranges from 0 to 20. This can be considered to be ordinal as a score of 0 indicates less function than a score of 20.

Figure 10.1 shows a histogram of these data. It shows that the distribution of the Barthel Index score at discharge is not Normal, with most of the participants scoring at the upper end of the scale, and only two participants scoring less than five. The distribution would undoubtedly be non-Normal if a histogram showing data by discharge destination was constructed, partly as a result of there being less data in the individual groups. Additionally, more than half of the participants scored between 15 and 20. This means that the independent samples t-test cannot be used and the Mann–Whitney U test should be used.

The specific null and alternative hypotheses for this example are:

H_0: There is no tendency for those who were discharged home to exceed those who were discharged to an institution in either direction in terms of the Barthel Index.

H_1: There is a tendency for those who were discharged home to exceed those who were discharged to an institution in either direction in terms of the Barthel Index.

To carry the Mann–Whitney U test out in SPSS go to Analyze → Nonparametric Tests → 2 Independent Samples…, where a dialog box like the one in Figure 10.2 will appear.

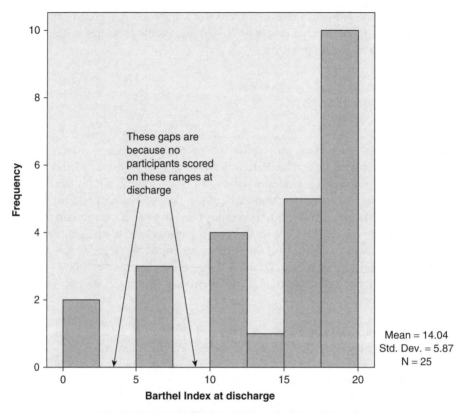

FIGURE 10.1   HISTOGRAM OF THE BARTHEL INDEX SCORE AT DISCHARGE (N=25)

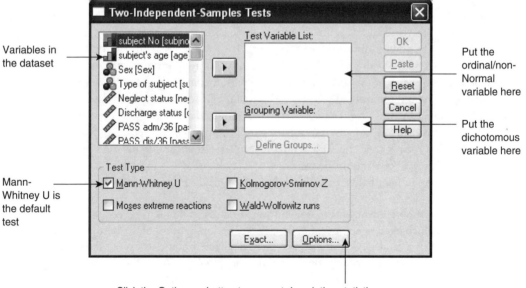

Click the Options… button to request descriptive statistics

FIGURE 10.2   TWO-INDEPENDENT-SAMPLES TESTS DIALOG BOX

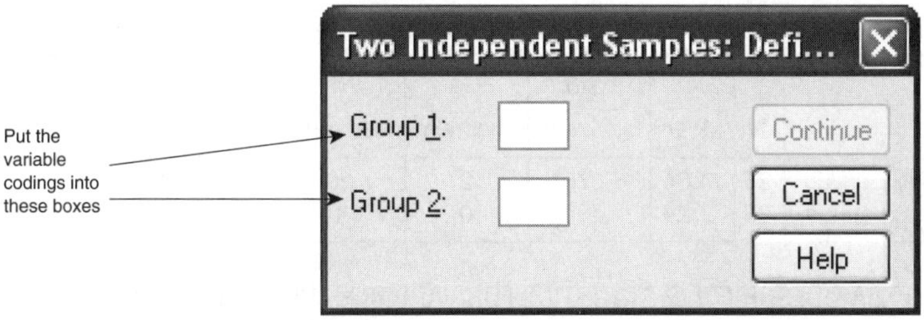

FIGURE 10.3   TWO INDEPENDENT-SAMPLES: DEFINE GROUPS DIALOG BOX

In the Two-Independent-Samples Tests dialog box (Figure 10.2), move the non-Normal (ordinal) variable to the Test Variable List: box and the dichotomous variable to the Grouping Variable: box. In the current example, the Test Variable is the Barthel Index at discharge and the Grouping Variable: is discharge status. As with the independent samples t-test the coding of the two groups (within discharge status) have to be defined by clicking on the Define Groups... button, where a dialog box like the one shown in Figure 10.3 is displayed. Put the coding for the two groups in the white boxes next to Group 1: and Group 2:. In this example the groups are coded 0 and 1. Coding can be checked using Variable View. When groups have been defined, click on Continue to return to the Two-Independent-Samples Tests dialog box (Figure 10.2).

From the Two-Independent-Samples Tests dialog box (Figure 10.2), click on the Options... button to get the dialog box in Figure 10.4. From this dialog box, tick Descriptive and Quartiles before clicking on the Continue button. Finally the OK button can be clicked on the Two-Independent-Samples Tests dialog box (Figure 10.2) to invoke the results (Figures 10.5a and 10.5b).

The test statistic for the Mann–Whitney U test is U. This is not usually reported in research papers, reports or dissertations. If U is very small then nearly all the first group is smaller than the second. If U is very large, then the converse is true, if U is moderate, then the groups are dispersed (and the result will not be significant). The

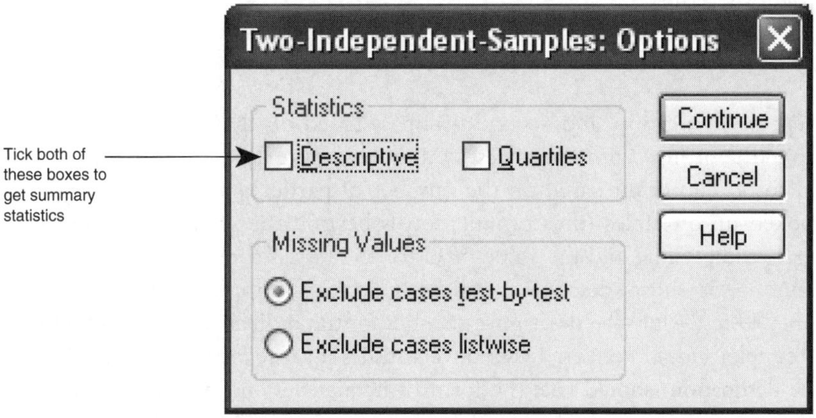

FIGURE 10.4   TWO-INDEPENDENT-SAMPLES: OPTIONS DIALOG BOX

Descriptive Stastistics

	N	Mean	Std. Deviation	Minimum	Maximum	Percentiles 25th	Percentiles 50th (Median)	Percentiles 75th
BARTHEL dis/20	25	14.04	5.870	2	20	10.50	16.00	19.00
Discharge status	25	.24	.436	0	1	.00	.00	.50

FIGURE 10.5A   DESCRIPTIVE STATISTICS FOR VARIABLES USED IN THE MANN-WHITNEY U TEST FOR THE BARTHEL INDEX AT DISCHARGE BY DISCHARGE STATUS

Ranks

	Discharge status	N	Mean Rank	Sum of Ranks
BARTHEL dis/20	Discharged home	19	15.71	298.50
	Discharged to an institution	6	4.42	26.50
	Total	25		

Test Statistics[b]

	BARTHEL dis/20	
Mann-Whitney U	5.500	← The test statistic U
Wilcoxon W	26.500	
Z	−3.293	
Asymp. Sig. (2-tailed)	.001	← This is the p-value associated with the Mann-Whitney U test
Exact Sig. [2*(1-tailed Sig.)]	.000[a]	

[a] Not corrected for ties
[b] Grouping Variable: Discharge status

FIGURE 10.5B   MANN-WHITNEY U TEST FOR THE BARTHEL INDEX AT DISCHARGE BY DISCHARGE STATUS

concept of 'first group' and 'second group' is based on the coding of the grouping variable (the groups with the lowest coding being the 'first group'). An upper value for U to be significant based on the number of participants in the two groups can be looked up on tables (the computation is beyond the scope of this book). SPSS will give the p-value and the value of U for the test as shown in Figure 10.5b.

Figure 10.5a shows descriptive statistics for the two variables used in the Mann-Whitney U test. Only the descriptive statistics for the ordinal variable (Barthel Index in this example) should be used. Descriptive statistics for categorical variables (such as discharge destination) should take the form of frequencies and percentages (as described previously in Chapter 6). As the Barthel Index is not Normally distributed in this dataset, the median and interquartile range (IQR) should be reported, and if there are a number of results given, they should be tabulated. The overall median Barthel Index score was 16

(IQR 10.5, 19.0). However, this may not be useful for presenting in a report, dissertation or thesis as it would be more useful to present summary statistics by group (discharge status in this example). These can be obtained using Explore (Chapter 5).

Interpretation

The Mann-Whitney test shown in the example in Figure 10.5b is statistically significant (p = 0.001), and therefore the null hypothesis can be rejected, showing a relationship between discharge status and Barthel Index score. The ranks can also be interpreted. From Figure 10.5b, it can be seen that there are mean ranks associated with both groups. The mean rank is much higher for those discharged home than those discharged to an institution, meaning that when the Barthel Index scores are ranked, on average those who were discharged home had a higher rank (indicating a higher Barthel Index score) than those who were discharged to an institution.

The differences between groups can be illustrated graphically using boxplots. Figure 10.6 shows Boxplots of the Barthel Index by discharge status (further details on boxplots are shown in Chapter 5). It shows that the median (and interquartile range) is much higher for those discharged home than those discharged to an institution (the same data as was shown in the descriptive statistics in Figure 10.5a). The boxplots also show there was one outlier in the group discharged to an institution (participant number 9) who had a much higher Barthel Index score (15) than others discharged to an institution.

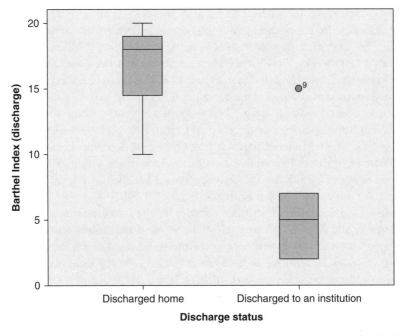

FIGURE 10.6   BOXPLOTS OF THE BARTHEL INDEX AT DISCHARGE BY DISCHARGE STATUS

KRUSKAL-WALLIS H TEST

The Kruskal-Wallis H test is an extension of the Mann-Whitney U test when there are three or more groups; so can be considered to be the non-parametric equivalent of the one-way analysis of variance (ANOVA). In common with other non-parametric tests the Kruskal-Wallis H test gives a p-value only. The general null and alternative hypotheses for this test are:

H_0: There is no difference in mean ranks between the groups studied.
H_1: There is a difference in mean ranks between the groups studied.

The Kruskal-Wallis test will be illustrated with the Barthel Index at hospital discharge and three patient groups; those with neglect that were discharged home; those without neglect that were discharged home and those with neglect who were discharged to an institution. This dataset also included one person without neglect, who was discharged to an institution. They were omitted from this analysis: they were filtered out using Select Cases (described in Chapter 2). The specific null and alternative hypotheses for this example are:

H_0: There is no difference in mean ranks between those without neglect discharged home, those with neglect discharged home, and those with neglect discharged to an institution.
H_1: There is a difference in mean ranks between those without neglect discharged home, those with neglect discharged home, and those with neglect discharged to an institution.

To invoke the Kruskal-Wallis H test in SPSS click on Analyze → Nonparametric Tests → K Independent Samples… to give the Tests for Several Independent Samples dialog box shown in Figure 10.7. Move the non-Normal (ordinal) variable into the Test Variable List: box. In this example that is the Barthel index score at discharge from hospital. Put the categorical variable in the Grouping Variable: box (Type of subject in this example). When the Grouping Variable: box has been filled, click the Define Range… button to give the dialog box shown in Figure 10.8. This should be filled with the minimum and maximum coding for the grouping (categorical) variable; this is 1 and 3 in the current worked example. Then click Continue to return to the Tests for Several Independent Samples dialog box (Figure 10.7). From here click on the Options… button to get the Several Independent Samples: Options dialog box (Figure 10.9). From this dialog box, tick both Descriptive and Quartiles to request summary statistics. Click Continue followed by OK on the Tests for Several Independent Samples dialog box (Figure 10.7) to generate output (shown in Figure 10.10).

Figure 10.10a shows the descriptive statistics for the two variables selected for this test. However, the type of summary statistics presented are inappropriate for categorical variables, so it is only appropriate to use the summary statistics for the ordinal or non-Normal variable (Barthel Index score at discharge in the example shown here). Summary statistics produced as part of this test are not broken down by group, so may be of limited use, and summary statistics by group may be more appropriate for presenting in a dissertation, report, thesis or paper. These can be gained using Explore (see Chapter 5 for information on how to do this). Overall, the median Barthel Index score at discharge was 16 (IQR 11, 19).

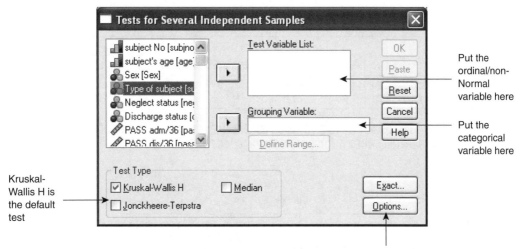

Tests for Several Independent Samples
subject No [subjno
subject's age [age]
Sex [Sex]
Type of subject [su
Neglect status [ne
Discharge status [c
PASS adm/36 [pa
PASS dis/36 [pass
Test Variable List:
Grouping Variable:
Define Range...
OK
Paste
Reset
Cancel
Help
Test Type
Kruskal-Wallis H
Median
Jonckheere-Terpstra
Exact...
Options...
Put the ordinal/non-Normal variable here
Put the categorical variable here
Kruskal-Wallis H is the default test
Click the Options… button to request descriptive statistics

FIGURE 10.7 TESTS FOR SEVERAL INDEPENDENT SAMPLES DIALOG BOX

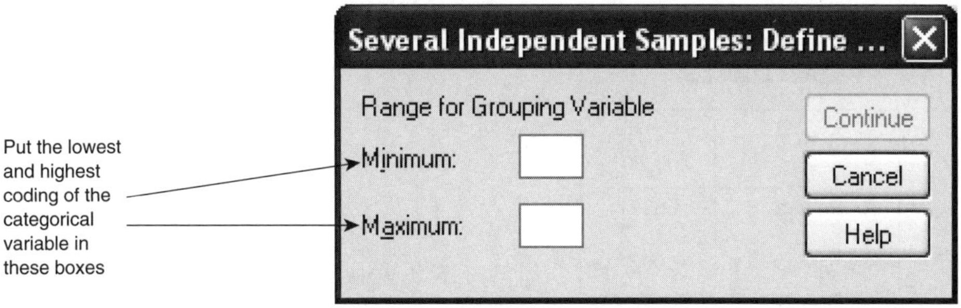

Several Independent Samples: Define ...
Range for Grouping Variable
Minimum:
Maximum:
Continue
Cancel
Help
Put the lowest and highest coding of the categorical variable in these boxes

FIGURE 10.8 SEVERAL INDEPENDENT SAMPLES: DEFINE RANGE DIALOG BOX

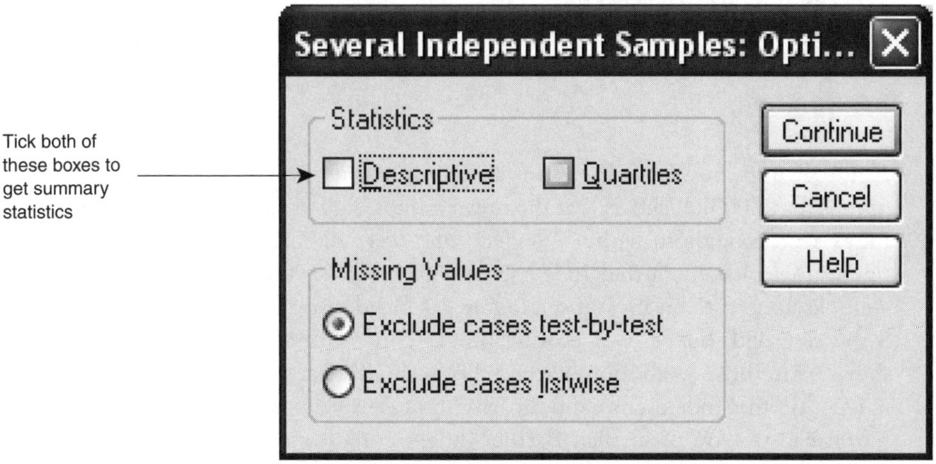

Several Independent Samples: Opti...
Statistics
Descriptive
Quartiles
Continue
Cancel
Help
Missing Values
Exclude cases test-by-test
Exclude cases listwise
Tick both of these boxes to get summary statistics

FIGURE 10.9 SEVERAL INDEPENDENT SAMPLES: OPTIONS DIALOG BOX

Descriptive Statistics

	N	Mean	Std. Deviation	Minimum	Maximum	Percentiles		
						25th	50th (Median)	75th
BARTHEL dis/20	24	14.42	5.679	2	20	11.25	16.00	19.00
Type of subject	24	1.92	.717	1	3	1.00	2.00	2.00

FIGURE 10.10A   DESCRIPTIVE STATISTICS FOR VARIABLES USED IN THE KRUSKAL-WALLIS H TEST FOR BARTHEL INDEX AT DISCHARGE BY NEGLECT AND DISCHARGE STATUS

Ranks

	Type of subject	N	Mean Rank
BARTHEL dis/20	subject with neglect home	7	11.50
	subject without neglect home	12	16.58
	subject with neglect to institution	5	4.10
	Total	24	

Test Statistics[a,b]

	BARTHEL dis/20
Chi-Square	11.321
df	2
Asymp. Sig.	.003

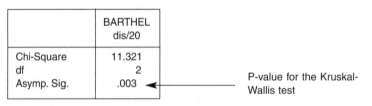

P-value for the Kruskal-Wallis test

[a] Kruskal-Wallis Test
[b] Grouping Variable: Type of subject

FIGURE 10.10B   KRUSKAL-WALLIS H TEST FOR BARTHEL INDEX AT DISCHARGE BY NEGLECT AND DISCHARGE STATUS

Interpretation

Figure 10.10b shows that there was a significant difference in the ranks of the three groups (p=0.003). It shows that the mean rank is highest (indicating a higher Barthel Index score) for those without neglect who were discharged home and the lowest (indicating a lower Barthel Index score) mean rank is for those with neglect who were discharged to an institution. Figure 10.11 goes some way to showing why this is the case with boxplots of Barthel Index score by discharge and neglect status. It shows that those without neglect who were discharged home had the highest median Barthel Index score, and those with neglect who were discharged to an institution had the lowest median Barthel Index score. Both of these discharge statuses had outliers; in the case of those discharged home without neglect, one participant

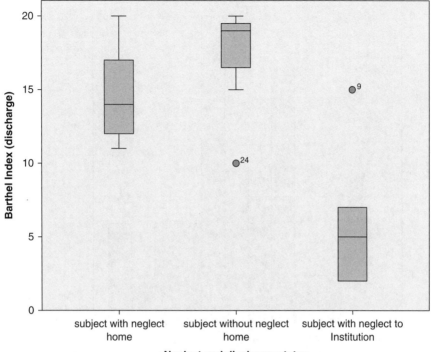

FIGURE 10.11   BOXPLOTS OF THE BARTHEL INDEX AT DISCHARGE BY NEGLECT AND DISCHARGE STATUS

had a score of 10 which was below the lower quartile, and in the case of those discharged to an institution with neglect one participant had a score above the upper quartile (these are identified by their study numbers in Figure 10.11).

WILCOXON MATCHED PAIRS TEST

This is a non-parametric analogue of the paired t-test, so can be used when the assumptions of the paired t-test are not met; chiefly that the differences between the data at the two time points are not Normally distributed. For this test to be valid the data must be interval (size of differences between values having a meaning). In addition, as with the paired t-test only participants with data present at both time points will be included in analysis and the variables of interest should be measuring the same thing which could be at different time points or under different conditions. The Wilcoxon matched pairs test provides a p-value only.

Null and alternative hypotheses for this test take the general form:

H_0: There is no tendency for one outcome to be higher or lower than the other.
H_1: There is a tendency for one outcome to be higher or lower than the other.

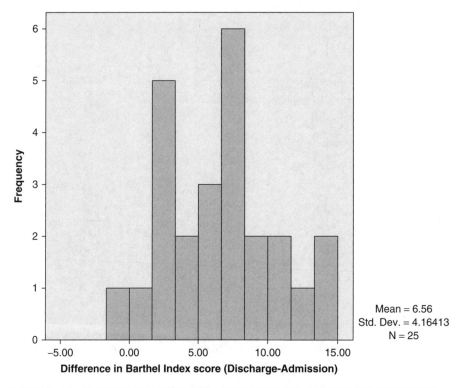

FIGURE 10.12   HISTOGRAM OF THE DIFFERENCE IN BARTHEL INDEX SCORE (DISCHARGE-ADMISSION)

This test ranks the differences between each matched pair (ignoring whether the differences are positive or negative at this point), so that the smaller differences are given smaller ranks and larger differences are given larger ranks. Where there are ties – that is, more than one difference of the same size – they are given ranks equal to the average of the ranks they would have received individually (and thus the same rank).

The Wilcoxon matched pairs test will be illustrated using the same dataset as used for the Mann-Whitney U test. This example will use the Barthel Index at admission to hospital and discharge from hospital. Figure 10.12 shows a histogram of the differences in Barthel Index score (discharge-admission). This is shown because an assumption of the paired t-test is that the differences are Normally distributed. Figure 10.12 shows that the data are not Normally distributed. This may be due to the size of the dataset, and that if the dataset was larger the differences may have been Normally distributed and parametric methods could have been used.

The specific null and alternative hypotheses for the Wilcoxon matched pairs test using these data are:

H_0: There is no tendency for the Barthel Index score at admission to be higher or lower than the Barthel Index score at discharge.

H_1: There is a tendency for the Barthel Index score at admission to be higher or lower than the Barthel Index score at discharge.

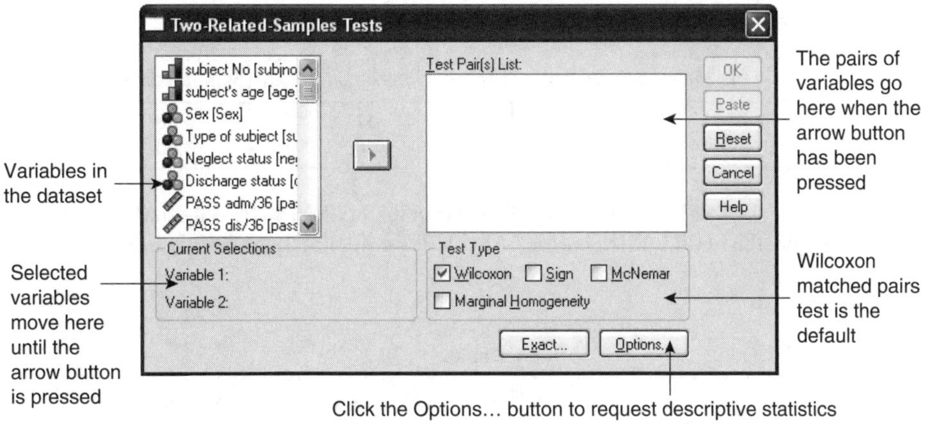

FIGURE 10.13   TWO-RELATED-SAMPLES TESTS DIALOG BOX

To do the Wilcoxon matched pairs test using SPSS, click on Analyze → Nonparametric Tests → 2 Related Samples… to give the dialog box shown in Figure 10.13. As with the paired t-test, two variables have to be selected by clicking on them. These will appear in the Current Selections box. When two variables are in the Current Selections box they can be moved to the Test Pair(s) List: box using the arrow. In the context of this example these are the Barthel Index score at admission to hospital and Barthel Index score at discharge from hospital. Following that click the Options… button to get a dialog box like the one shown in Figure 10.14. From this dialog box, tick Descriptive and Quartiles to obtain summary statistics. Then click Continue to return to the Two Related Samples Tests dialog box (Figure 10.13) then click OK to generate the output (Figures 10.15a and 10.15b).

Interpretation

Figure 10.15a shows the descriptive statistics for the Barthel Index at the two time points. The median score at admission to hospital was 6 (IQR 4, 12), whilst the median was 16 at discharge (IQR 10.5, 19.0). Figure 10.15b gives the results

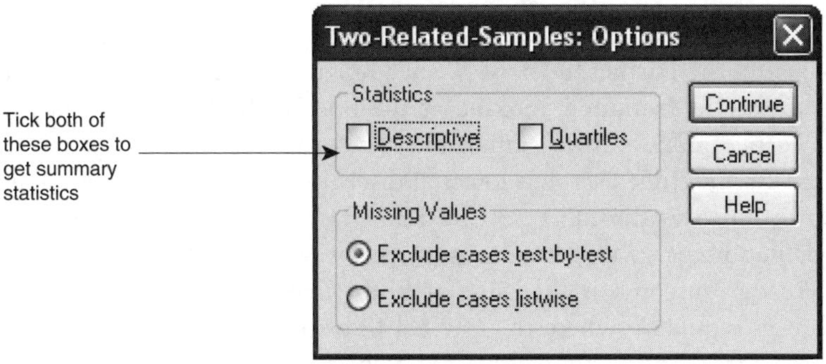

FIGURE 10.14   TWO-RELATED-SAMPLES: OPTIONS DIALOG BOX

Descriptive Stastitics

	N	Mean	Std. Deviation	Minimum	Maximum	25th	50th (Median)	75th
							Percentiles	
BARTHEL ad/20	25	7.48	4.968	0	17	4.00	6.00	12.00
BARTHEL dis/20	25	14.04	5.870	2	20	10.50	16.00	19.00

FIGURE 10.15A   DESCRIPTIVE STATISTICS FOR VARIABLES USED IN THE WILCOXON MATCHED PAIRS TEST FOR BARTHEL INDEX AT HOSPITAL ADMISSION AND DISCHARGE

Ranks

		N	Mean Rank	Sum of Ranks
BARTHEL dis/20 -BARTHEL ad/20	Negative Ranks	1[a]	1.50	1.50
	Positive Ranks	24[b]	13.48	323.50
	Ties	0[c]		
	Total	25		

[a] BARTHEL dis/20 < BARTHEL ad/20
[b] BARTHEL dis/20 > BARTHEL ad/20
[c] BARTHEL dis/20 = BARTHEL ad/20

Test Statistics[b]

	BARTHEL dis/20- BARTHEL ad/20
Z	−4.336[a]
Asymp. Sig. (2-tailed)	.000

The p-value for the Wilcoxon matched pairs test. A p-value given as 0.000 should be presented as p<0.001

[a]Based on negative ranks.
[b]Wilcoxon Signed Ranks Test.

FIGURE 10.15B   WILCOXON MATCHED PAIRS TEST FOR BARTHEL INDEX AT HOSPITAL ADMISSION AND DISCHARGE

of the Wilcoxon matched pairs test. It shows that there is a significant difference in the ranks of the Barthel Index between admission and discharge (p < 0.001). The ranks can also be examined; looking at the box labelled Ranks (Figure 10.15b), shows negative ranks, positive ranks and ties. In this example, negative ranks are where the Barthel Index score is lower at discharge than at admission. One partici-pant was in this situation. The positive ranks were where the Barthel Index score was higher at discharge than at admission, this was the case for 24 participants. Ties are where the outcome is the same at both time points; in the context of this example this would be where the Barthel Index score was the same at both time points. No participants scored the same at both time points. Therefore it can be seen that with the exception of one participant, all improved in terms of their Barthel Index score between admission and discharge.

SIGN TEST

The sign test is another non-parametric analogue of the paired t-test. Its general null and alternative hypotheses are:

H_0: The difference in score or value is equally likely to be positive or negative.
H_1: The difference in score or value is not equally likely to be positive or negative.

The sign test proceeds by calculating the difference in score between the two time points. Those observations where there is no difference (that is, scored the same at both time points, also called ties) are dropped from the analysis because they add no information regarding differences. If the null hypothesis were true, the number of positive and negative differences would be equal. The p-value is calculated using the binomial distribution, the derivation of which is beyond the scope of this book. SPSS gives the p-value for the test, which should be reported along with appropriate summary statistics (median and interquartile range or range for both time points or conditions). The sign test is illustrated using the same data as for the Wilcoxon matched pairs test; namely, Barthel Index at admission and discharge from hospital. The specific null and alternative hypotheses for this test and dataset are:

H_0: The differences in Barthel Index scores between discharge from hospital and admission to hospital are equally likely to be positive or negative.
H_1: The differences in Barthel Index scores between discharge from hospital and admission to hospital are not equally likely to be positive or negative.

The sign test in SPSS is invoked in the same way as the Wilcoxon matched pairs test; that is, by clicking on Analyze → Nonparametric Tests → 2 related samples…, giving the dialog box in Figure 10.13. In this dialog box, the Wilcoxon matched pairs test should be unticked and the Sign ticked. Click the Options… button on the Two Related Samples Tests dialog box (Figure 10.13) to get the Two Related Samples: Options dialog box (Figure 10.14) where Descriptive and Quartiles should be ticked, then click Continue followed by OK. The results from this analysis can be seen in Figure 10.16. This shows that there was strong evidence that the differences in Barthel Index scores are not equally likely to be positive or negative ($p < 0.001$). The box containing the frequencies show the numbers of participants that had differences in Barthel Index scores (discharge-admission). The negative differences are where the Barthel Index at discharge is lower than that at admission. This was the case for one participant. The positive differences are where the Barthel Index score is higher at discharge than admission ($n = 24$). There were no participants who scored the same on the Barthel Index at admission and discharge. If there had been, these would have been omitted from this sign test analysis.

Frequencies

		N
BARTHEL dis/20	Negative Differences[a]	1
-BARTHEL ad/20	Positive Differences[b]	24
	Ties[c]	0
	Total	25

[a]BARTHEL dis/20 < BARTHEL ad/20
[b]BARTHEL dis/20 > BARTHEL ad/20
[c]BARTHEL dis/20 = BARTHEL ad/20

Test Statistics[b]

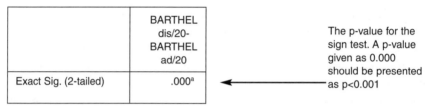

	BARTHEL dis/20- BARTHEL ad/20
Exact Sig. (2-tailed)	.000[a]

The p-value for the sign test. A p-value given as 0.000 should be presented as p<0.001

[a]Binomial distribution used.
[b]Sign Test.

FIGURE 10.16   RESULTS OF THE SIGN TEST FOR BARTHEL INDEX AT HOSPITAL ADMISSION AND DISCHARGE

Note: descriptive statistics and quartiles for the sign test have been suppressed in Figure 10.16 because they are the same as those presented in Figure 10.15.

WHICH TEST IS 'BETTER', WILCOXON MATCHED PAIRS TEST OR SIGN TEST?

It is clear that the Wilcoxon matched pairs test has the advantage of using more data than the sign test, as the Wilcoxon matched pairs test uses all data regardless of whether a difference has been shown between variables; that is, data with ties are included. This is potentially very important in a dataset that has a large number of differences of zero, meaning that a lot of data would be dropped with the sign test. It is important to analyse those who show no difference as well as those who show positive or negative differences. As more data are used with the Wilcoxon matched pairs test than the sign test, it would usually be expected that the Wilcoxon matched pairs test will give a smaller p–value (more significant result). Looking at the example shown in this chapter comparing the Barthel Index at admission and discharge, as there were no ties, and there was only one negative rank (difference), both tests gave the same result, with a p–value of <0.001.

FRIEDMAN'S TEST

Friedman's test is an extension of the Wilcoxon matched pairs test for situations where there are more than two time points. Therefore, only those participants who have data present at all time points are included in analysis. As with other non-parametric tests, this is a hypothesis test only, meaning that only a p-value is given as the result of the test. The general null and alternative hypotheses for Friedman's test are:

H_0: There is no difference in mean ranks between time points or conditions tested.

H_1: There is a difference in mean ranks between time points or conditions tested.

For this example the same dataset will be used; however, this time the outcome of interest will be the Postural Assessment Scale for Stroke (PASS) (Benaim et al., 1999), which assesses balance and posture in people who have had a stroke. The maximum possible score on this measure is 36, whilst the minimum is 0. This measure will be used for this example because assessment was carried out at three time points: admission to hospital, discharge from hospital and five weeks post discharge. The specific null and alternative hypotheses for this example are:

H_0: There is no difference in mean ranks between PASS scores at admission, discharge and post discharge.

H_1: There is a difference in mean ranks between PASS scores at admission, discharge and post discharge.

To invoke Friedman's test in SPSS, click on Analyze → Nonparametric Tests → K Related Samples.... This will give the dialog box shown in Figure 10.17. Move the three or more variables which give the scores at three or more time points to the Test Variables: box. Using the PASS example at three time points, PASS score at

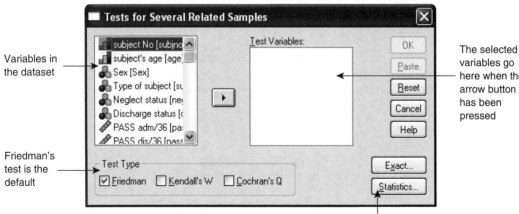

Click the Statistics... button to request descriptive statistics

FIGURE 10.17   SEVERAL RELATED SAMPLES TESTS DIALOG BOX

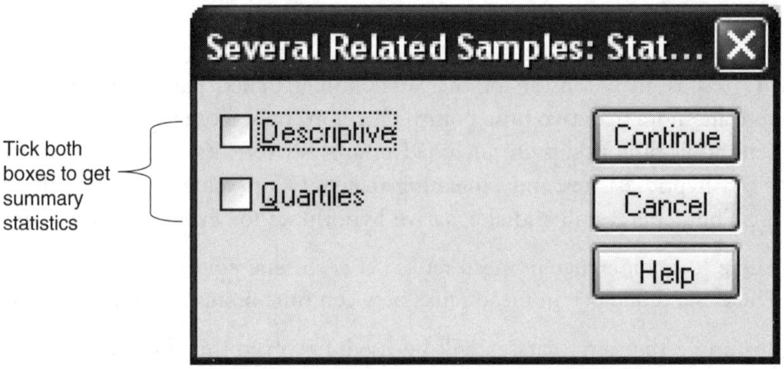

FIGURE 10.18   SEVERAL RELATED SAMPLES: STATISTICS DIALOG BOX

admission, discharge and post discharge should be moved to the Test Variables: box. Then, click the Statistics… button to give the Several Related Samples: Statistics dialog box shown in Figure 10.18. From this dialog box, tick Descriptive and Quartiles for summary statistics of the data. Then click Continue to return to the Tests for Several Related Samples dialog box (Figure 10.17) then click OK to give the output (Figures 10.19a and 10.19b).

Interpretation

Figure 10.19a shows that 25 participants completed the assessment at the three time points. The median score on the PASS improved with increasing time since stroke, with the median at admission being 10 (IQR 1.5, 26.0) compared to 27 (IQR 14, 32) at discharge and 30 (IQR 16.0, 31.5) at five weeks post discharge. Friedman's test was highly significant ($p < 0.001$) (Figure 10.19b).

SUMMARY

- Non-parametric tests are used when the assumptions of parametric tests are not met.
- The Mann-Whitney U test is the non-parametric equivalent of the independent sample t-test. In SPSS it can be invoked by going to Analyze → Nonparametric Tests → 2 Independent Samples… .

Descriptive Statistics

	N	Mean	Std. Deviation	Minimum	Maximum	Percentiles		
						25th	50th (Median)	75th
PASS adm/36	25	13.16	11.316	1	30	1.50	10.00	26.00
PASS dis/36	25	23.08	10.785	1	35	14.00	27.00	32.00
PASS post did/36	25	23.72	12.050	1	35	15.00	30.00	31.00

FIGURE 10.19A   DESCRIPTIVE STATISTICS FOR VARIABLES USED IN FRIEDMAN'S TEST FOR PASS AT HOSPITAL ADMISSION, DISCHARGE AND POST-DISCHARGE

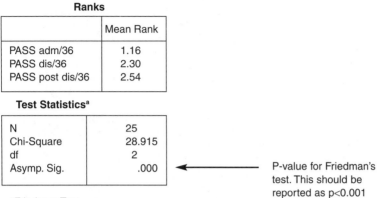

Ranks

	Mean Rank
PASS adm/36	1.16
PASS dis/36	2.30
PASS post dis/36	2.54

Test Statistics[a]

N	25
Chi-Square	28.915
df	2
Asymp. Sig.	.000

P-value for Friedman's test. This should be reported as $p<0.001$

[a]Friedman Test

FIGURE 10.19B   FRIEDMAN'S TEST FOR PASS AT HOSPITAL ADMISSION, DISCHARGE AND POST-DISCHARGE

- The Kruskal-Wallis H test is an extension of the Mann-Whitney U test. To use it in SPSS click on Analyze → Nonparametric Tests → K Independent Samples… .
- The Wilcoxon matched pairs test and sign test are both non-parametric equivalents of the paired t-test. Using SPSS they can be employed by clicking on Analyze → Nonparametric Tests → 2 related samples… .
- Friedman's test is an extension of the Wilcoxon matched pairs test. In SPSS it can be used by clicking on Analyze → Nonparametric Tests → K Related Samples… .

EXERCISES

Table 10.1 shows outcomes one year after stroke, comparing conventional treatment with the intervention treatment (Rudd et al., 1997). Look at the Table and answer the questions that follow.

TABLE 10.1   OUTCOMES ONE YEAR AFTER STROKE IN A RANDOMISED CONTROLLED TRIAL COMPARING COMMUNITY THERAPY AND CONVENTIONAL THERAPY

Variable	Community therapy	Conventional	P-value
Barthel Index			
Mean (SD)	16 (4)	16 (4)	
Median (range)	18 (2–20)	18 (3–20)	0.30
Number assessed	135	126	

(Continued)

(Continued)

Five-metre timed walk			
Mean seconds (SD)	12 (6)	12 (8)	
Median seconds (range)	10 (6–40)	9 (6–70)	0.34
Number assessed	99	90	
Total Nottingham health profile			
Mean (SD)	14 (9)	12 (8)	
Median (range)	13 (0–42)	12 (0–36)	0.11
Number assessed	118	105	
Rivermead activities of daily living scale			
Mean (SD)	27 (12)	27 (11)	
Median (range)	25 (15–45)	25 (15–45)	0.93
Number assessed	132	121	
Caregiver strain			
Mean (SD)	5 (4)	4 (3)	
Median (range)	5 (0–12)	3 (0–12)	0.14
Number assessed	75	59	

1 What statistical tests were used to assess differences between community therapy and conventional therapy?
2 How would you interpret the results of the five-metre timed walk as presented in Table 10.1?
3 Using the results given, what would you conclude?

In a quasi experimental study comparing people with hand injuries receiving origami therapy with those receiving usual care only, it was found that the median change in seconds in the Jebsen-Taylor Hand Function Test between baseline and the end of the study was 11.8 (range 1.2, 69.2) for the origami group and 4.3 (range –2.6, 9.0) for the usual care group, $p = 0.06$. (Wilson et al., 2008)

4 Which test has been used to generate these results?
5 What do you notice about the statistics for those who received usual care?
6 How would you interpret a p-value of 0.06?

Open smoking.sav.

7 Investigate the relationship between age at which the participant started smoking and their gender. You may find it useful to construct histograms or a box and whisker plot of the data before deciding which test to do. Which test did you use? What does the statistical test show?
8 Using the same dataset, determine whether there is an association between current age group in three categories (up to 34 years, 35–44 years and 45+ years) and age at which they started smoking. Which test was used? Was it statistically significant?

11
ASSESSING ASSOCIATIONS WITH A CONTINUOUS OUTCOME

INTRODUCTION

When analysing continuous variables, sometimes the analysis requires that the relationship between them is examined to see how closely they are related to one another. Initially, this can be done visually using a scatterplot. If the relationship is shown to be linear, correlations can be done to indicate the strength and direction of the relationship between the two variables in question. If the assumptions of Pearson's product moment correlation – a parametric test, are violated, there is a non-parametric equivalent which can be used instead.

Once it has been established that there is a linear relationship between the two variables in question, it is possible to discover how much one variable changes in relation to the other variable, this is termed simple linear regression. However, in most situations there may be more than one factor related to the outcome. Possible associations of this kind can be assessed with an extension of simple linear regression – multiple linear regression. This chapter also explains two-way analysis of variance (ANOVA), showing its relationship with multiple linear regression.

The data for the worked examples in this chapter come from the student obesity study.

THE AIMS OF THIS CHAPTER ARE:

- To plot data using SPSS to show visually the relationship between two continuous variables.
- To learn about correlation; what it means, when to use it and how to do it in SPSS.
- To explain simple linear regression and how to invoke it in SPSS.
- To extend the principles of simple linear regression to multiple linear regression.
- To look at two-way ANOVA; its uses and how to employ SPSS to calculate it.

CORRELATION

Correlation is used to discover how closely related to one another two variables are. There are two forms that will be considered in this chapter, the parametric version, called Pearson's product moment correlation (usually referred to as Pearson's correlation) and the non-parametric equivalent: Spearman's rank correlation.

PEARSON'S PRODUCT MOMENT CORRELATION

This is what people usually mean when they refer to correlation (if they have not mixed up the terms correlation and association). It measures the strength and direction of a linear association between two continuous variables. It does not measure causation, so that if a strong correlation has been found, it does not mean that one variable causes the other. Depending on the variables in question this may not make clinical sense either. For example, if the variables being correlated are measures of well-being, then one variable could not possibly cause the other.

For Pearson's correlation to be valid data should be independent of one another. In its simplest form, this means that there should only be one set of data from each participant. Additionally, at least one variable per correlation must be Normally distributed. This assumption should be tested using histograms of the variables. Histograms are explained further in Chapter 5. If variables are not Normally distributed, it may be possible to transform them by taking logarithms or the square root of the data. If this is not possible, use Spearman's rank correlation described later in this chapter.

Once it has been established that at least one variable to be analysed is Normally distributed, it is important to plot the variables against one another using a scatterplot to check whether the relationship between the variables is linear. Variables may have a non-linear relationship with one another (for example quadratic, like the one shown in Figure 11.1). If this is the case, Pearson's correlation will not correctly indicate the strength of the relationship.

Interpretation

From Figure 11.1, it can be seen that there is a strong (near perfect) inverse quadratic relationship between these two measures of lung function. The Pearson's correlation coefficient for these data is −0.896, which although strong does not reflect the strength of non-linear relationship shown by the scatterplot.

Plotting two continuous variables

The example used for the next part of this chapter is the student obesity data. It was established in Chapter 5 that the distribution of height is Normally distributed. Weight will be the other continuous variable used.

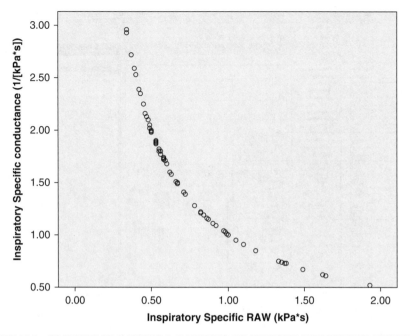

FIGURE 11.1   SCATTERPLOT SHOWING A QUADRATIC RELATIONSHIP BETWEEN TWO MEASURES OF LUNG FUNCTION IN ONE-YEAR-OLD CHILDREN WHO WERE BORN EXTREMELY PRETERM

To invoke scatterplots in SPSS, click Graphs → Chart Builder… where the same dialog box as shown in Figure 5.1 (Chapter 5) is shown. From the list of graph types to choose from, click on Scatter/Dot then drag the graphic style shown in the top left of the style gallery (Simple Scatter) to the large white box in the upper half of the dialog box. When this has been completed, the dialog box changes to that shown in Figure 11.2.

Now drag height and weight from the Variables: list to the x-Axis? and y-Axis? boxes respectively. Add titles if required by clicking on the Titles/Footnotes tab on the Chart Builder then typing the required title into the appropriate space in the Element Properties dialog box. Then click OK to produce the graph shown in Figure 11.3.

Interpretation

Figure 11.3 shows the height and weight of each participant with data for both variables. Each participant is represented by a circle on the graph, with some circles overlapping where participants are the same height and weight. The data from the participants in the upper box are worth noting; these are heavier than most participants of a similar height. In contrast, those in the lower box are lighter than participants of a similar height. The data points in the boxes should be borne in mind when the correlation is carried out, since outliers influence the correlation coefficient.

The pattern produced by Figure 11.3 shows that generally, as height increases, weight increases too. This is characterised by the pattern of data points going from the bottom left of the scatterplot to the top right. That means, in this dataset, generally taller people weigh more than shorter people. Therefore, this relationship is positive linear.

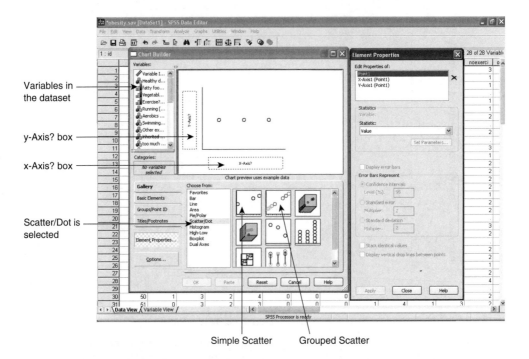

Variables in the dataset

y-Axis? box

x-Axis? box

Scatter/Dot is selected

Simple Scatter   Grouped Scatter

FIGURE 11.2   CHART BUILDER DIALOG BOX WITH SCATTERPLOT SELECTED

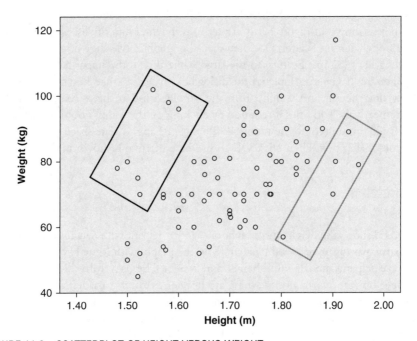

FIGURE 11.3   SCATTERPLOT OF HEIGHT VERSUS WEIGHT

Another point to note is that there may be a different relationship between the two variables between underlying groups. For example, the pattern of height and weight may be different by sex. A scatterplot in SPSS to show this can be created by

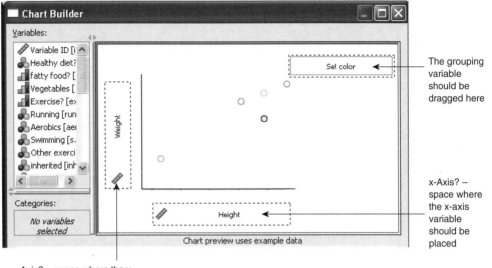

The grouping variable should be dragged here

x-Axis? – space where the x-axis variable should be placed

y-Axis? – space where the y-axis variable should be placed

FIGURE 11.4   UPPER PORTION OF THE CHART BUILDER DIALOG BOX SHOWING GROUPED SCATTER

dragging the Grouped Scatter graph style (indicated in Figure 11.2) to the large box at the top of the Chart Builder dialog box, which will then look like Figure 11.4.

Drag the grouping variable (sex in this example) to the Set color box, make sure the two continuous variables (height and weight in this example) have been dragged to the x-Axis? and y-Axis? places. Then click OK to give the scatterplot shown in Figure 11.5.

Interpretation

Figure 11.5 shows data for females and males. It shows that generally males are taller and heavier than females. The relationship between height and weight appears to be similar for the sexes, with the females forming the lower portion and males forming the upper portion. In this circumstance it is acceptable to correlate data for males and females combined. However, if further analyses are carried out, gender may be a significant factor in explaining height or weight.

Back to Pearson's correlation

Pearson's correlation coefficient is denoted by r. It can take any value between −1 and +1. Where the correlation coefficient is −1 to 0, this indicates a negative correlation such that as one variable increases the other decreases. On a scatterplot this is shown by the data points going from top left to bottom right. A perfect negative correlation is shown with a correlation coefficient of −1. Where the correlation coefficient is 0 to +1, this is a positive correlation (as shown in Figures 11.3 and 11.5 with data points going from bottom left to top right), such that as one variable increases in magnitude, the

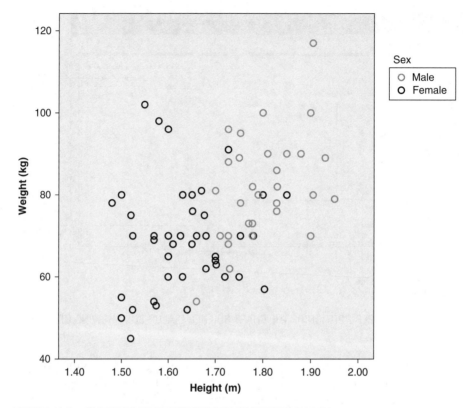

FIGURE 11.5   SCATTERPLOT OF HEIGHT VERSUS WEIGHT BY SEX

other one does too. A perfect positive correlation is denoted by a correlation coefficient of +1. Where the correlation coefficient is 0, no correlation is indicated, and no discernable pattern of data points will be apparent on a scatterplot. An example of such a relationship can be seen later in this chapter in Figure 11.12.

It is possible to do significance tests on correlations, with the general null and alternative hypotheses being:

H$_0$: There is no linear relationship between the two continuous variables of interest in the population. This equates to the true population correlation coefficient being zero.

H$_1$: There is a linear relationship between the two continuous variables of interest in the population.

These equate to the specific hypotheses using the current variables of:

H$_0$: There is no linear relationship between height and weight in the population.

H$_1$: There is a linear relationship between height and weight in the population.

The test statistic (which is beyond the scope of this book) follows a t-distribution with n−2 degrees of freedom. SPSS will give the resulting p-value, but not the test

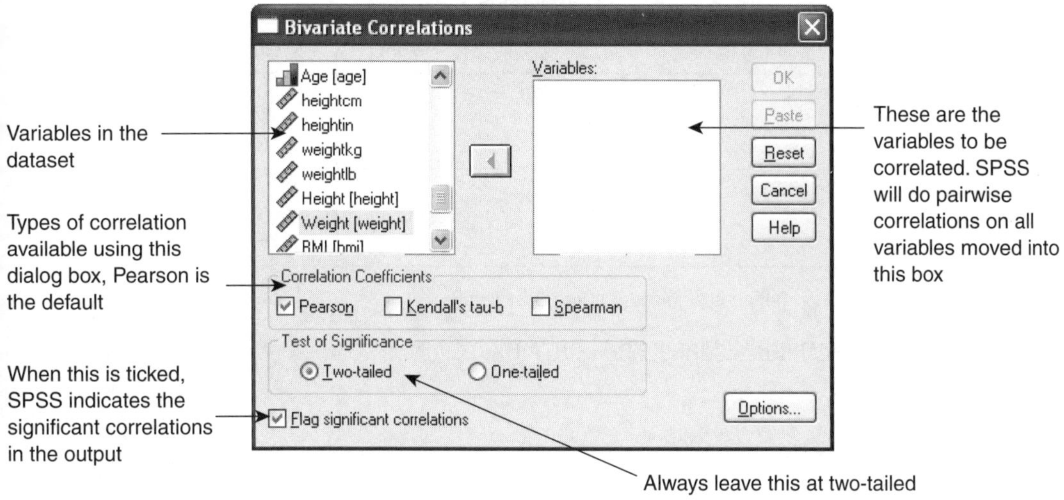

Variables in the dataset

Types of correlation available using this dialog box, Pearson is the default

When this is ticked, SPSS indicates the significant correlations in the output

These are the variables to be correlated. SPSS will do pairwise correlations on all variables moved into this box

Always leave this at two-tailed

FIGURE 11.6   BIVARIATE CORRELATIONS DIALOG BOX

statistic. The test statistic for Pearson's correlation is not reported in papers or reports. If p<0.05 (statistically significant), it is concluded that data are not consistent with the null hypothesis and conclude that the true correlation coefficient in the population is not zero, meaning there is a linear relationship between the two variables in question. The significance test only tells whether there is a real relationship, not the strength of the relationship. The strength of the relationship is given by the correlation coefficient r. This means that the strength of relationship as defined by r may not be high, but the significance test may indicate a highly significant finding. This is especially important to bear in mind as the lower limit for the correlation coefficient to be significant decreases with increasing sample size. For example, if there were 30 participants in the dataset, the lower limit of correlation coefficient to be significant is $r = \pm0.36$, whereas if there were 100 participants this decreases to $r = \pm0.20$ (Bland, 2000); neither of these are considered to be strong correlations.

Confidence intervals can also be constructed for correlation coefficients as long as both variables are Normally distributed. However, the underlying mathematics is complex, and SPSS does not calculate these statistics. For information on how to calculate 95% confidence intervals for correlation coefficients see Bland (2000).

To carry out Pearson's correlation using SPSS, click on Analyze $\rightarrow$ Correlate $\rightarrow$ Bivariate... to give the dialog box shown in Figure 11.6.

Move the required variables (at least two variables) into the Variables: box; in this example height and weight will be used. Then click OK to give the output shown in Figure 11.7. It is possible to move as many variables as desired to the Variables: box and SPSS will calculate all pairwise correlations between the variables selected, regardless of whether the assumptions of Pearson's correlation have been met. They are outputted to a correlation matrix (a larger version of Figure 11.7 containing all pairwise correlations requested).

Correlations

		Height	Weight
Height	Pearson Correlation	1	.440**
	Sig. (2-tailed)		.000
	N	76	73
Weight	Pearson Correlation	.440**	1
	Sig. (2-tailed)	.000	
	N	73	76

**. Correlation is significant at the 0.01 level

FIGURE 11.7   PEARSON'S CORRELATION OUTPUT

Interpretation

Figure 11.7 shows the correlation between height and weight. In each cell of the table there is the Pearson's correlation coefficient, the two sided p-value and the number of participants' data used to calculate the correlations. It can be seen that the correlations between height and height and between weight and weight are 1. This means that the correlation between these is perfect positive linear, which is to be expected, if a scatterplot of height versus height (using the same data) was to be constructed, it would show a straight line of observations from bottom left to top right. Moving to the correlations between height and weight, it can be seen these are shown twice – in the bottom left and top right of the output. When reporting correlations in papers, reports or dissertations, it is usual to only report the correlations in the lower half of the table, as those in the upper half of the table use the same data as those in the lower half. The correlation coefficient between height and weight of 0.44 shows a moderate positive correlation (as shown visually in Figure 11.3), with a p-value of <0.001. The p-value indicates that the correlation coefficient of 0.44 is significantly different to 0.

SPEARMAN'S RANK CORRELATION

If the assumption of normality is not met, making the use of Pearson's correlation not possible, it is possible to use Spearman's rank correlation instead. This is the non-parametric analogue of Pearson's correlation. It should be used where both variables are ordered or when both variables are not Normally distributed and cannot be transformed. As with other non-parametric methods, Spearman's rank correlation is based upon ranking the data (ordering it) rather than the actual values of the data. Therefore, plotting the data on a scatterplot is unlikely to give an indication of the relationship between the variables.

The correlation coefficient is denoted by rho (ρ) and can take any value between −1 and +1, with a similar interpretation to that of Pearson's correlation. Likewise, significance tests can be carried out on Spearman's rank correlation with null hypothesis and alternative hypotheses taking the general form:

H_0: There is no relationship between the two variables in question.
H_1: There is a relationship between the two variables in question (either one variable increases as the other increases or one variable increases as the other decreases).

Spearman's rank correlation is invoked in SPSS in the same way as Pearson's correlation, namely by clicking on Analyze → Correlate → Bivariate... when the dialog box shown in Figure 11.6 appears, untick Pearson and tick Spearman to indicate the type of correlation required. The output from SPSS appears to be identical to that of Pearson's correlation in presentation.

For example, Mussaffi et al., (2007) used Spearman's rank correlation to correlate children's and caregivers' responses on asthma specific quality of life measures. The measure for the caregivers measured their quality of life in relation to the child's condition. Spearman's rank correlation was used because both scales were ordered (1 to 7, where 1 = low quality of life) and neither were Normally distributed. In addition, the correlation between the child's quality of life measure and asthma severity score (1 = mild asthma, 4 = severe asthma) was examined. The study found that $\rho = 0.61$ ($p < 0.001$) for the correlation between children's and caregivers' quality of life score, indicating a strong positive relationship between children's and their caregivers' perception of quality of life. This was statistically significant, indicating the correlation was different from zero. This was in contrast to the correlation between asthma severity and children's quality of life score, where $\rho = 0.17$ ($p > 0.05$). As the p-value was greater than 0.05 a correlation different from zero has not been shown (consistent with the null hypothesis).

SIMPLE LINEAR REGRESSION

Having found a linear correlation between two continuous variables using Pearson's correlation, it is often useful to be able to predict one variable from the other or discern the magnitude of influence one variable has over the other. This can be done using regression, as the primary aim of regression is to assess the nature rather than the strength of a relationship. The variable that is being predicted is called the response, outcome or dependent variable. The variable that is used to explain the relationship also has a number of names: explanatory, predictor or independent variable. Here, the terms dependent and independent variables will be used to be consistent with the terminology used in SPSS.

The general null and alternative hypotheses for each independent variable (separately) are:

H_0: There is no linear relationship between the dependent variable and the independent variable in question.
H_1: There is a relationship between the dependent variable and the independent variable in question.

There are assumptions associated with simple linear regression. The first is that there should be a linear relationship between the two variables. Secondly, the values of the dependent variable should be Normally distributed for each value of the independent variable and that the variance (standard deviation) should be the same at each of these points. Finally, the observations should be independent of one another. If each observation does not originate from a different person, simple linear regression (or multiple linear regression shown later in this chapter) should not be used. Apart from the final assumption, ways to check these are shown later in this chapter. If the assumptions are not met, it may be possible to transform the data. However, interpretation is more complex if one or more variables are transformed.

Simple linear regression is solved using the method of least squares giving an equation $y = a + \beta x$ where y is the dependent variable and x is the independent variable. α is the intercept (sometimes called the constant), that is the point at which the independent variable $x = 0$. This is often a theoretical concept, for example, if we consider weight = y and height = x, the situation where height = 0 is impossible, so extrapolation should not extend beyond the range of the data available. This value is rarely reported in papers, theses, dissertations or reports unless the regression line and equation are shown on a scatterplot. β is the slope (sometimes called gradient); that is, the increase in the dependent variable (y) when the independent variable (x) increases by one unit.

One of the statistics that is produced when linear regression is calculated is R^2. In linear regression this is the correlation coefficient r (which is also given in the output) squared. This is interpreted as the amount of variation that is explained by the variables in the model, ranging from 0 to 1 (but can be multiplied by 100 so that it can be expressed as a percentage). The difference between 1 and the reported R^2 will come from variables not in the model (which there may or may not be data in the dataset on). However, R^2 should not be used as an indicator of the model fit since it generally increases with increasing numbers of variables in the model, regardless of whether they are significant or not.

Simple linear regression will be illustrated using the same height and weight variables previously utilised, weight will be the dependent variable and height will be the independent variable. To invoke simple linear regression in SPSS click Analyze → Regression → Linear... to get the dialog box shown in Figure 11.8.

In terms of the obesity data, the aim is to discover the relationship between weight and height, with weight being the dependent variable. Therefore, weight is put in the box labelled Dependent:. Height is placed in the box labelled Independent(s):. The most appropriate method of model selection is Enter, which is also the default. It is then necessary to click on the Statistics... button to give the dialog box in Figure 11.9. From Figure 11.9 the Confidence intervals box should be ticked, the default (as shown in Figure 11.9) is not to give confidence intervals for the regression coefficient. However, as it was discussed in Chapter 7, it is important to present 95% confidence intervals in papers, reports, or dissertations where possible, often in preference to p-values. In the context of linear regression coefficients, 95% confidence intervals that do not include 0 (whether they are positive or negative) indicate a statistically significant coefficient.

Descriptive statistics (mean, standard deviation and Pearson's correlations) can also be requested from the Linear Regression: Statistics dialog box by ticking the box next to Descriptives. When all statistics have been requested, click Continue to return to the Linear Regression dialog box (Figure 11.8).

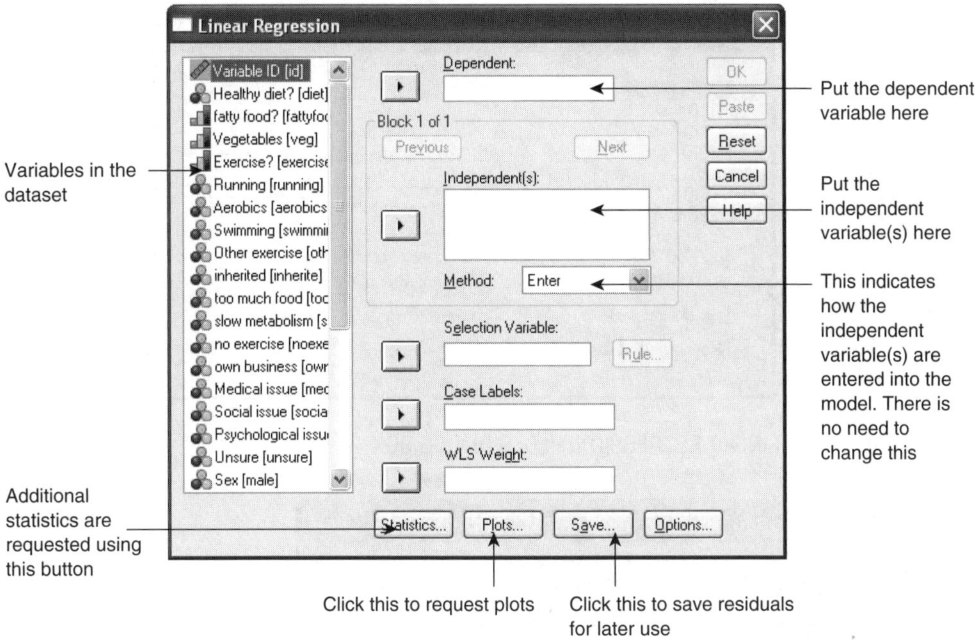

Variables in the dataset

Additional statistics are requested using this button

Put the dependent variable here

Put the independent variable(s) here

This indicates how the independent variable(s) are entered into the model. There is no need to change this

Click this to request plots

Click this to save residuals for later use

FIGURE 11.8 THE LINEAR REGRESSION DIALOG BOX

Tick this box to get confidence intervals for the regression coefficient

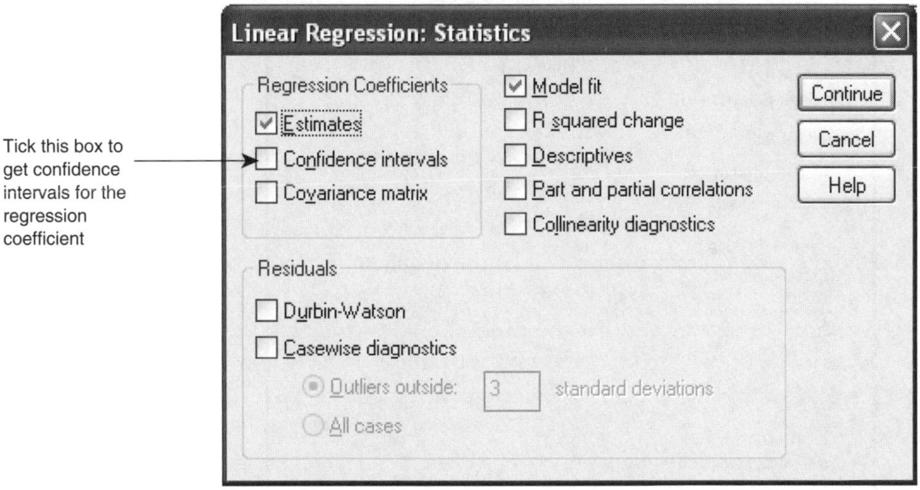

FIGURE 11.9 LINEAR REGRESSION: STATISTICS DIALOG BOX

Next on the Linear Regression dialog box click on the Plots… button to give the dialog box in Figure 11.10. Plots are constructed to check the assumptions of simple linear regression. The most appropriate plots to request are: a histogram of the standardised residuals or a Normal probability plot of residuals. The histogram of residuals and normal probability plot can be requested by ticking the boxes next to Histogram and Normal probability plot.

When the required plots have been selected, click Continue to return to the Linear Regression dialog box (Figure 11.8). Finally, click the Save… button to give the dialog

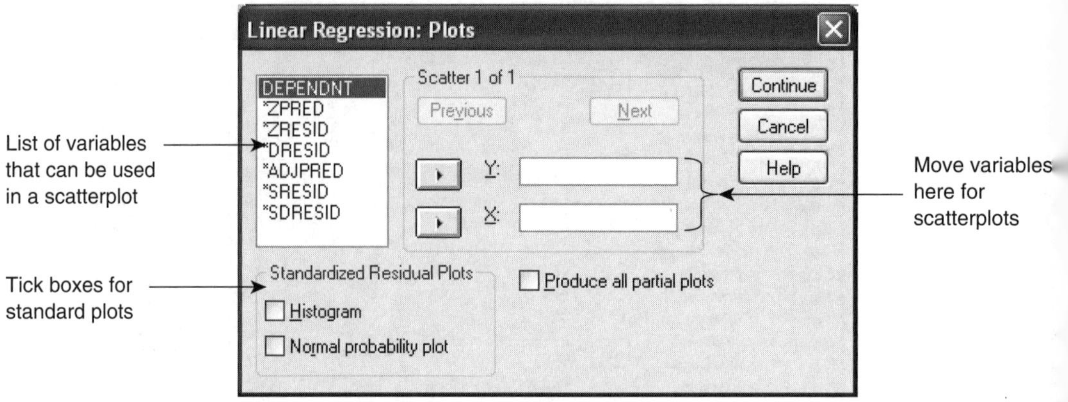

List of variables that can be used in a scatterplot

Move variables here for scatterplots

Tick boxes for standard plots

FIGURE 11.10   LINEAR REGRESSION: PLOTS DIALOG BOX

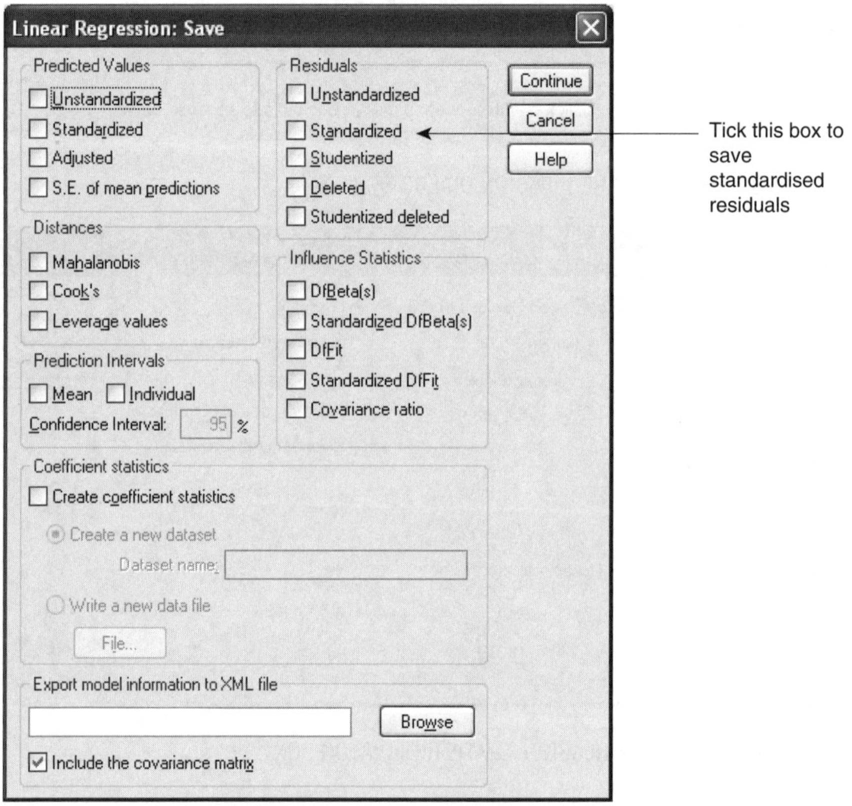

Tick this box to save standardised residuals

FIGURE 11.11   LINEAR REGRESSION: SAVE DIALOG BOX

box shown in Figure 11.11. From this dialog box, tick the Standardized Residuals box so they can be used later. Then click Continue to return to the Linear Regression dialog box (Figure 11.8) before clicking OK to give the output shown in Figure 11.13.

It was shown earlier in this chapter using a scatterplot that there was a linear relationship between height and weight in this dataset (Figure 11.3). To check the assumption

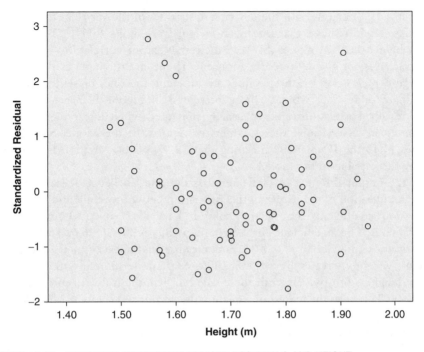

FIGURE 11.12   SCATTERPLOT OF STANDARDISED RESIDUALS AND HEIGHT

of the dependent variable being Normally distributed for each value of the independent variable, the standardized residuals (saved to the dataset whilst executing simple linear regression; the variable appears at the far right of the dataset) should be plotted on a histogram to ensure there is a Normal distribution with a mean of 0. To check that the variance of the dependent variable is constant across differing values of the independent variable, a scatterplot (details of how to do this are shown earlier in this chapter) of the standardised residuals versus the independent variable should be constructed. If the assumption holds, there should be no relationship between the standardised residuals and independent variable. To confirm this, the Pearson's correlation can be checked; and the correlation coefficient (r) should be close to 0.00. The scatterplot of the standardised residuals and height is shown in Figure 11.12.

Interpretation

Figure 11.12 shows a scatterplot of the standardised residuals versus height (the independent variable), this shows there is no relationship between these two variables ($r=0.00$) so the assumption of the variance of the independent variable being constant across values of the independent variable, and the regression analysis is valid. Likewise the assumption of Normally distributed residuals was fulfilled as shown by the histogram of residuals and the Normal probability plot shown in Figure 11.13. In order to indicate that the residuals are Normally distributed, the Normal probability plot should show data in a straight line from bottom left to top right. The one shown in Figure 11.13 shows a slight deviation, but is acceptable.

Figure 11.13 begins with the descriptive statistics of the variables that are used in this model. It shows that the mean weight was 74.6kg (SD 14.2kg) and the mean height was 1.71 metres (SD 0.12 metres). Next the correlations between the two variables are given, the correlation coefficients are the same as those shown in Figure 11.7, however, the p-values are different; the ones presented in Figure 11.13 are one sided, whereas those presented in Figure 11.7 are two sided. Additionally, correlations are not usually presented when linear regressions are presented in dissertations, theses, papers or reports. In the Model Summary of Figure 11.13 the R^2 is 0.194 meaning that 19.4% of the variation is accounted for by the variable in the model.

In the output the next box of interest is the one labelled Coefficients. These give an indication of the nature of the association between weight and height. The regression coefficients are in the column labelled B under Unstandardized Coefficients. The coefficient for height is 51.35 (95% CI 26.6, 76.1). This is statistically significant ($p < 0.001$). This means that for every metre increase in height, weight increases by 51.35kg. The constant term refers to the weight when height is 0m (which, with these data is a hypothetical concept). This value is -12.99. This gives the regression equation of: weight $= -12.99 + (51.35 \times$ height). The histogram shows that the standardised residuals can be considered to be Normally distributed, which is confirmed by looking at the Normal probability plot (Figure 11.13).

Descriptive Statistics

	Mean	Std. Deviation	N
Weight	74.64	14.157	73
Height	1.7065	.12135	73

Correlations

		Weight	Height
Pearson Correlation	Weight	1.000	.440
	Height	.440	1.000
Sig. (1-tailed)	Weight		.000
	Height	.000	
N	Weight	73	73
	Height	73	73

Be aware that the p-values shown here are for a one sided test. P-values for two sided tests can be obtained using the Bivariate Correlations dialog box

Variables Entered/Removed[b]

Model	Variables Entered	Variables Removed	Method
1	Height[a]		Enter

[a]All requested variables entered.
[b]Dependent Variable: Weight

(Continued)

FIGURE 11.13 *(Continued)*

Model Summary[b]

Model	R	R Square	Adjusted R Square	Std. Error of the Estimate
1	.440[a]	.194	.182	12.081

[a]Predictors: (Constant), Height
[b]Dependent Variable: Weight

R^2 for this model

ANOVA[b]

Model		Sum of Squares	df	Mean Square	F	Sig.
1	Regression	2795.844	1	2795.844	17.061	.000[a]
	Residual	11634.896	71	163.872		
	Total	14430.740	72			

[a]Predictors: (Constant), Height
[b]Dependent Variable: Weight

Coefficients[a]

Model		Unstandardized Coefficients		Standardized Coefficients	t	Sig.	95% Confidence Interval for B	
		B	Std. Error	Beta			Lower Bound	Upper Bound
1	(Constant)	−12.990	21.269		−.611	.543	−55.400	29.419
	Height	51.353	12.433	.440	4.131	.000	26.563	76.143

[a]Dependent Variable: Weight

Beta coefficient for height

p-value for height, this should be presented as p<0.001

95% C1 for around the beta coefficient for height

Residuals Statistics[a]

	Minimum	Maximum	Mean	Std. Deviation	N
Predicted Value	63.01	87.15	74.64	6.231	73
Residual	−22.619	35.424	.000	12.712	73
Std. Predicted Value	−1.867	2.007	.000	1.000	73
Std. Residual	−1.767	2.767	.000	.993	73

[a]Dependent Variable: Weight

(Continued)

(Continued)

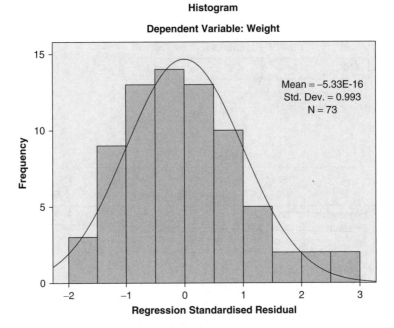

Histogram

Dependent Variable: Weight

Mean = −5.33E-16
Std. Dev. = 0.993
N = 73

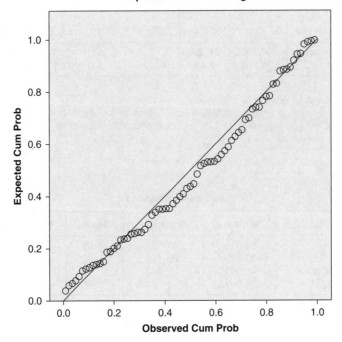

Normal P-P Plot of Regression Standardised Residual

Dependent Variable: Weight

FIGURE 11.13   SIMPLE LINEAR REGRESSION OF WEIGHT AND HEIGHT OUTPUT

MULTIPLE LINEAR REGRESSION

Simple linear regression can be extended to include more than one independent variable, which could be continuous, categorical or a mixture of both. The regression equation can also be extended to include the additional factors in the model. For example, Figure 11.4 indicates that sex of the participant may be important in determining weight as it shows that males tend to be heavier than females. Linear regression using more than one independent variable is called multiple linear regression. Multiple linear regression is invoked in the same way as simple linear regression: namely, by clicking Analyze → Regression → Linear... to give the dialog box shown in Figure 11.7.

As with simple linear regression, the dependent variable should be transferred to the Dependent: box. Independent variables are then transferred to the Independent(s): box. For those variables with two categories it is beneficial to code the categories 0 and 1 so that the category coded 0 is the comparison category. If categorical variables with more than two categories are included in the regression model, SPSS expects these as dummy variables. For example, to add age group, in the form of a dummy variable (an explanation of dummy variables and how to create them is given in Chapter 2) as an independent variable in multiple linear regression, the variables Age3140 and Age4150 would have to be transferred to the Independent(s): box shown in Figure 11.7.

To enable the user to have most control over the modelling process, it is advisable to retain Enter as the Method:. This means that all variables will be entered and retained in the model and the user can then decide which variables are removed from the model. This is especially important where there are dummy variables because if another model selection technique (such as stepwise, forwards or backwards) was used SPSS may exclude one of the dummy variables because it is not significant; if at least one dummy variable representing part of a variable with more than two categories (such as Age3140, Age4150 representing agegroup) is significant then all dummy variables relating to that variable should be retained.

An example of multiple linear regression output is shown in Figure 11.14 using weight as the dependent variable, with height and sex as the independent variables.

Interpretation

Before starting the main interpretation, note that the descriptive statistics for sex (Figure 11.14) should not be presented as it is nonsensical to present a mean for a categorical variable. Likewise, if correlations are requested, beware that the p-values shown are for one sided tests, whereas in health statistics the results of two sided significance tests should be presented unless there is a good, justifiable reason to do otherwise. It can also be seen that the standardised residuals (shown in the histogram at the end of Figure 11.14) do not appear to be perfectly Normal, however bearing in mind the size of the dataset and the general trend of the residuals exhibited, this is acceptable.

Descriptive Statistics

	Mean	Std. Deviation	N
Weight	74.64	14.157	73
Height	1.7065	.12135	73
Sex	.42	.498	73

Correlations

		Weight	Height	Sex
Pearson Correlation	Weight	1.000	.440	.436
	Height	.440	1.000	.702
	Sex	.436	.702	1.000
Sig. (1-tailed)	Weight	.	.000	.000
	Height	.000	.	.000
	Sex	.000	.000	.
N	Weight	73	73	73
	Height	73	73	73
	Sex	73	73	73

Variables Entered/Removed[b]

Model	Variables Entered	Variables Removed	Method
1	Sex, Height[a]		Enter

[a]All requested variables entered.
[b]Dependent Variable: Weight

Model Summary

Model	R	R Square	Adjusted R Square	Std. Error of the Estimate
1	.475[a]	.225	.203	12.637

[a]Predictors: (Constant), Sex, Height

ANOVA[b]

Model		Sum of Squares	df	Mean Square	F	Sig.
1	Regression	3252.617	2	1626.309	10.184	.000[a]
	Residual	11178.123	70	159.687		
	Total	14430.740	72			

[a]Predictors: (Constant), Sex, Height
[b]Dependent Variable: Weight

(Continued)

FIGURE 11.14   *(Continued)*

Coefficients[a]

Model		B	Std. Error	Beta	t	Sig.	Lower Bound	Upper Bound
		Unstandardized Coefficients		Standardized Coefficients			95% Confidence Interval for B	
1	(Constant)	18.907	28.223		.670	.505	−37.381	75.195
	Height	30.893	17.233	.265	1.793	.077	−3.476	65.262
	Sex	7.106	4.201	.250	1.691	.095	−1.274	15.485

[a]Dependent Variable: Weight

Residuals Statistics[a]

	Minimum	Maximum	Mean	Std. Deviation	N
Predicted Value	64.63	86.25	74.64	6.721	73
Residual	−23.295	35.227	.000	12.460	73
Std. Predicted Value	−1.490	1.727	.000	1.000	73
Std. Residual	−1.843	2.788	.000	.986	73

[a]Dependent Variable: Weight

Charts

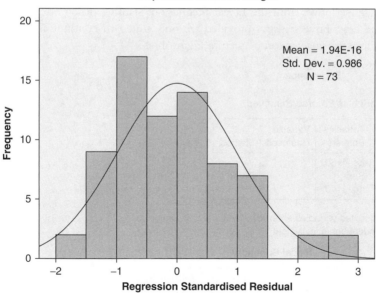

Histogram

Dependent Variable: Weight

Mean = 1.94E-16
Std. Dev. = 0.986
N = 73

FIGURE 11.14   MULTIPLE LINEAR REGRESSION WITH ONE CONTINUOUS AND ONE CATEGORICAL INDEPENDENT VARIABLE OUTPUT

The mean weight was 75kg (SD 14kg), whilst the mean height was 1.71m (SD 0.12m). Males were on average 7.1kg (95% CI −1.3, 15.5) heavier than females, however, this is not statistically significant (p = 0.095). Lack of statistical significance can also be seen by looking at the 95% CI, which includes 0, the null value. Twenty-three per cent of the variation in the data was accounted for by the model.

In the output shown in Figure 11.14, neither height nor sex was statistically significant, so if this was to be presented the least significant of the two variables (sex in this case) would be removed and the model refitted (to give output the same as shown in Figure 11.13) unless it had been decided a priori to control for demographic factors such as sex.

MULTIPLE LINEAR REGRESSION WITH TWO CATEGORICAL INDEPENDENT VARIABLES

The final multiple linear regression example to be shown is one where both independent variables are categorical; here the dependent variable is weight and the independent variables are sex and age group in three categories. The category representing the lowest age group (ages 11 to 30 years) is the comparison category. Remember when including a categorical variable with more than two categories these should be entered as dummy variables. In this example there are two dummy variables, age3140 representing those aged 31 to 40 years and age4150 representing those aged 41+. The procedure for obtaining multiple linear regression output with two categorical variables is the same as shown earlier in this chapter, although it should be noted that it does not make sense to select Descriptives from the Linear Regression: Statistics dialog box (Figure 11.9), since the descriptive statistics provided are only suited to continuous variables. The output from this analysis can be seen in Figure 11.15.

Regression

Variables Entered/Removed[b]

Model	Variables Entered	Variables Removed	Method
1	age4150, Sex, age3140[a]		Enter

[a]All requested variables entered.
[b]Dependent Variable: Weight

Model Summary

Model	R	R Square	Adjusted R Square	Std. Error of the Estimate
1	.433a	.187	.154	13.035

[a]Predictors: (Constant), age4150, Sex, age3140

(Continued)

FIGURE 11.15   (*Continued*)

ANOVA[b]

Model		Sum of Squares	df	Mean Square	F	Sig.
1	Regression	2821.181	3	940.394	5.535	.002[a]
	Residual	12233.555	72	169.910		
	Total	15054.737	75			

[a]Predictors: (Constant), age4150, Sex, age3140
[b]Dependent Variable: Weight

Coefficients[a]

Model		Unstandardized Coefficients		Standardized Coefficients	t	Sig.	95% Confidence Interval for B	
		B	Std. Error	Beta			Lower Bound	Upper Bound
1	(Constant)	69.528	2.991		23.245	.000	63.566	75.491
	Sex	12.297	3.042	.431	4.042	.000	6.233	18.361
	age3140	.273	3.581	.010	.076	.939	−6.866	7.412
	age4150	−.347	4.029	−.011	−.086	.932	−8.378	7.684

[a]Dependent Variable: Weight

FIGURE 11.15   MULTIPLE LINEAR REGRESSION WITH TWO CATEGORICAL INDEPENDENT VARIABLES OUTPUT

Interpretation

Analysis shown in Figure 11.15 shows that males are on average 12.3kg (95% CI 6.2kg, 18.4kg) heavier than females whilst controlling for age group. Age group is not significantly associated with weight of participant. In this example, the constant represents the average weight of females aged less than 31 years old. This is because females and those aged less than 31 years are the comparison categories for sex and age respectively.

As with the previous example which showed non-significant variables, it would be usual to remove the variable that is least significant unless it had been decided a priori to control for that factor. It is also necessary to remember that if it is decided to remove age group from the analysis, both dummy variables (in the example shown in Figure 11.15 this would be age3140 and age4150) must be removed else the model will not make sense. Additionally, as was shown earlier in this chapter the model which includes sex is also not significant, and if sex is removed, the model (using these data) reverts back to that of simple linear regression.

TWO-WAY ANALYSIS OF VARIANCE (ANOVA)

This is an extension of the one-way ANOVA shown in Chapter 9. Instead of including one independent factor as with one-way ANOVA, it includes two independent factors (categorical variables). Using this procedure will give the same ANOVA p-values as multiple linear regression; giving the overall p-value for factors with more than two categories. Two-way ANOVA will not give beta coefficients so it is not possible to attribute an effect size to the result. To invoke two-way ANOVA in SPSS click on Analyze → General Linear Model → Univariate… to give a dialog box as shown in Figure 11.16. The dependent variable should be continuous.

Using the obesity data previously used to illustrate linear regression, sex and age of the participants will be examined; both of these should be placed in the Fixed Factor(s): box in the Univariate dialog box whilst weight, as the dependent variable should be placed in the Dependent Variable: box (Figure 11.16). Unlike multiple linear regression, ANOVA is able to accept categorical variables with more than two categories as they are entered into SPSS (that is, there is no need to make dummy variables).

Then, from the right hand side of the Univariate dialog box click Options…, which will give the dialog box shown in Figure 11.17. In this dialog box tick Descriptive statistics, this will give descriptive statistics (mean, SD and N) by the two factors in the analysis. If descriptive statistics are required for within each factor then the two factors shown in the Factor(s) and Factor Interactions: box should be transferred to the Display Means for: box. Then click Continue to return to the Univariate dialog box (Figure 11.16).

When setting up a two-way ANOVA (or extensions thereof), the default is to carry out a full factorial model. This is one that includes the individual factors as well as an interaction term; that is, looking to see whether the effect of one categorical variable in the model is changed by the presence of another variable in the model. Interactions are explained further by Altman and Matthews (1996). However, there is no justification to do this unless the presence of an interaction has been hypothesised before analysing the data. Models can become more complex when they are extended further to include more than two categorical variables as all possible combinations of interactions are computed. With many interactions interpretation may become difficult. Therefore the type of model has to be changed. To do this, click the Model… button on the Univariate dialog box (Figure 11.16) to give the Univariate: Model dialog box (Figure 11.18). Under Specify Model, select the Custom radio button. This will allow the options under Build Term(s) to be changed; change it to Main Effects so that no interactions are computed. Then select the variables listed under Factors & Covariates: and transfer them to the Model: box. Then click Continue to return to the Univariate dialog box (Figure 11.16), then click OK to give the output (the output for the example described here is shown in Figure 11.19).

Interpretation

The greatest mean weight was in men aged 41 years and over at 84.3kg (SD 14.1kg), conversely women aged over 40 years had the lowest mean weight at 67.3kg (SD 13.8kg). It was found that there was no significant effect of age group ($p = 0.986$) on weight, whilst sex was statistically significant ($p < 0.001$).

As with the analogous multiple linear regression, it may be felt that there is no justification in retaining age group in the analysis as it was not statistically significant, if this was the case the analysis would revert back to a one-way ANOVA as there would only be one independent variable remaining in the model.

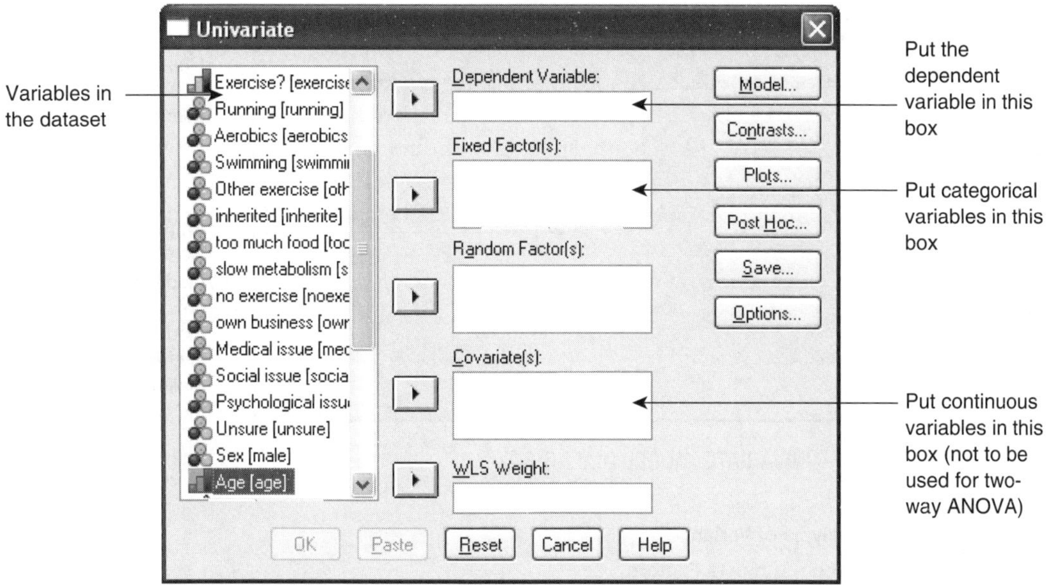

Variables in the dataset

Put the dependent variable in this box

Put categorical variables in this box

Put continuous variables in this box (not to be used for two-way ANOVA)

FIGURE 11.16   UNIVARIATE DIALOG BOX

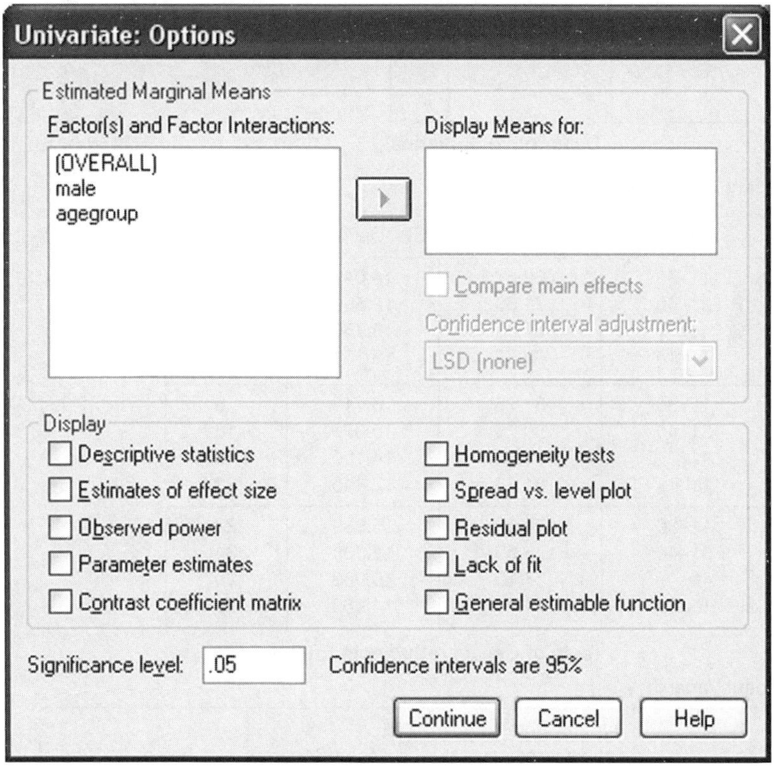

FIGURE 11.17   UNIVARIATE: OPTIONS DIALOG BOX

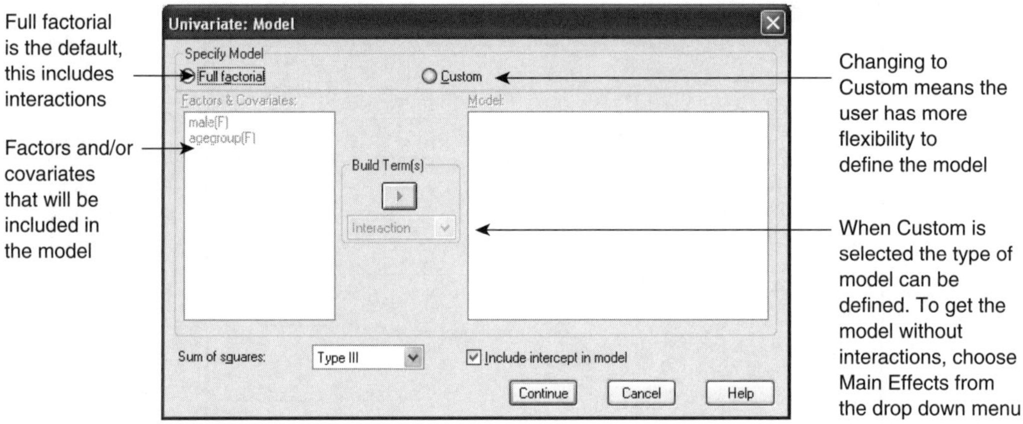
Full factorial is the default, this includes interactions
Factors and/or covariates that will be included in the model
Univariate: Model
Specify Model
Full factorial
Custom
Factors & Covariates:
male(F)
agegroup(F)
Build Term(s)
Interaction
Model:
Sum of squares:
Type III
Include intercept in model
Continue
Cancel
Help
Changing to Custom means the user has more flexibility to define the model
When Custom is selected the type of model can be defined. To get the model without interactions, choose Main Effects from the drop down menu

FIGURE 11.18 UNIVARIATE: MODEL DIALOG BOX

Univariate Analysis of Variance

Between-Subjects Factors

		Value Label	N
Sex	0	Female	44
	1	Male	32
Age group	1	11–30	22
	2	31–40	34
	3	41+	20

Descriptive Statistics

Dependent Variable: Weight

Sex	Age group	Mean	Std. Deviation	N
Female	11–30	69.57	14.042	14
	31–40	71.00	12.589	18
	41+	67.33	13.760	12
	Total	69.55	13.151	44
Male	11–30	81.75	16.113	8
	31–40	80.75	10.070	16
	41+	84.25	14.130	8
	Total	81.88	12.445	32
Total	11–30	74.00	15.639	22
	31–40	75.59	12.334	34
	41+	74.10	15.983	20
	Total	74.74	14.168	76

Tests of Between-Subjects Effects

Dependent Variable: Weight

Source	Type III Sum of Squares	df	Mean Square	F	Sig.
Corrected Model	2821.181[a]	3	940.394	5.535	.002
Intercept	400185.683	1	400185.683	2355.274	.000

(*Continued*)

FIGURE 11.19   (*Continued*)

Source	Type III Sum of Squares	df	Mean Square	F	Sig.
male	2776.480	1	2776.480	16.341	.000
agegroup	4.854	2	2.427	.014	.986
Error	12233.555	72	169.910		
Total	439560.000	76			
Corrected Total	15054.737	75			

[a]R Squared = .187 (Adjusted R Squared = .154)

Estimated Marginal Means

Sex

Dependent Variable: Weight

Sex	Mean	Std. Error	95% Confidence Interval	
			Lower Bound	Upper Bound
Female	69.504	1.981	65.555	73.452
Male	81.801	2.359	77.099	86.502

FIGURE 11.19   TWO-WAY ANOVA OUTPUT

SUMMARY

- Scatterplots are used to visually explore the relationship between two continuous variables. They can be invoked using Graphs → Chart Builder... .
- Pearson's product moment correlation can be used to show the strength and direction of a relationship between two variables where at least one variable is Normally distributed. In SPSS the command sequence is Analyze → Correlate → Bivariate... .
- Where the assumptions of the Pearson's product moment correlation are violated, Spearman's correlation can be used. The command sequence in SPSS is the same as for Pearson's product moment correlation.
- Simple linear regression is used to determine the nature of a relationship between two continuous variables. It can also be used to predict the values of one variable from the other. It can be invoked in SPSS by clicking on Analyze → Regression → Linear... .
- Multiple linear regression is an extension of simple linear regression which allows more independent variables, which can be continuous or categorical, to be included. It is invoked in the same way as simple linear regression in SPSS.
- Two-way ANOVA is initiated in SPSS by clicking on Analyze → General Linear Model → Univariate... .

EXERCISES

Table 11.1 shows Pearson's correlation coefficients of the Bayley MDI (Bayley, 1993) and parent report measures. Linguistic skills comprise vocabulary and sentence complexity. Parent report composite comprises non-verbal cognition, vocabulary and sentence complexity.

TABLE 11.1   PEARSON'S CORRELATION COEFFICIENTS BETWEEN PARENT REPORTED COGNITIVE SCORES AND MDI* SCORES

Measure	(1)	(2)	(3)	(4)	(5)	(6)
MDI (1)	1.00					
Non-verbal cognition (2)	0.54	1.00				
Vocabulary (3)	0.63	0.53	1.00			
Sentence complexity (4)	0.67	0.66	0.78	1.00		
Linguistic skills (5)	0.66	0.57	0.99	0.84	1.00	
Parent report composite (6)	0.68	0.67	0.98	0.86	0.99	1.00

*Mental Development Index from the Bayley Scales of Infant Development (Bayley, 1993)

Source: Johnson et al., 2004: 391

1   What is the Pearson's correlation coefficient for MDI and linguistic skills?
2   Interpret the correlation coefficient for MDI and linguistic skills in terms of its strength and direction.
3   Why are the correlation coefficients for linguistic skills and vocabulary and linguistic skills and sentence complexity so high?

The following extract and Table 11.2 come from a four year study of people who were 85 years old at recruitment. The study measure, depressive symptoms and cognitive function over time.

> … Correlation between depressive symptoms and cognitive function at baseline. Depressive symptoms were significantly correlated with lower scores for global cognitive function, attention, processing speed, and immediate and delayed recall and with higher test scores for attention (indicating reduced attention) (all $P < 0.001$). (Vinkers et al., 2004)

TABLE 11.2   CROSS SECTIONAL CORRELATION OF DEPRESSIVE SYMPTOMS* WITH VARIOUS MEASURES OF COGNITIVE FUNCTION IN 500 PEOPLE AGED 85 YEARS LIVING IN THE COMMUNITY

Cognitive function test	Pearson's correlation coefficient (r)	p-value
Global cognitive function	−0.296	<0.001
Attention	0.182	<0.001
Processing speed	−0.238	<0.001
Immediate recall	−0.194	<0.001
Delayed recall	−0.182	<0.001

*Depressive symptoms assessed with the 15 item geriatric depression scale (GDS-15)

Source: Vinkers et al., 2004: 882

4   What does a p-value <0.001 mean in relation to correlation (as shown in Table 11.2)?

5   Why is the correlation so low (r) yet the p-value indicates high significance?

Look at the regression coefficients shown in Table 11.3 and answer the questions. The dependent variable is the number of words children born extremely preterm can vocalise using a standardised tool at two years old.

TABLE 11.3   RESULTS OF MULTIPLE LINEAR REGRESSION TO DETERMINE FACTORS AFFECTING NUMBER OF WORDS VOCALISED

Independent variable	Beta coefficient	95% confidence interval
Age at time outcome was measured (years)	58.04	(30.68, 85.39)
Female sex	Reference	
Male sex	−10.01	(−16.08, −3.94)
Length of hospital stay (days)	−0.16	(−0.26, −0.06)
Standardised weight at 12 months	3.58	(1.20, 5.96)
No disability	Reference	
Mild disability	−10.53	(−17.22, −3.83)
Severe disability	−25.52	(−36.59, −14.45)

Source: Marston et al., 2009

6   If they were not statistically significant, which variables might have been included in the model regardless?

7   Which variables shown in Table 11.3 are categorical?

8   Interpret the coefficients for sex and number of days spent in hospital.

12

ASSESSING ASSOCIATIONS WITH A CATEGORICAL OUTCOME

INTRODUCTION

Chapter 11 looked at situations where the dependent variable is continuous and explained a number of statistical techniques which can be used with such data. However, not all dependent variables are continuous, meaning those methods are not appropriate in those circumstances. For example, the outcome may be whether a participant has a specific type of cancer; the dependent variable would be yes (cancer present) versus no (cancer not present). This chapter starts by returning to the concept of probability by putting it into practice in order to calculate odds and odds ratios from cross tabulations. From this, SPSS is used to show how to obtain the same odds ratio, and also the 95% confidence interval. Finally logistic regression is introduced; which in its simplest form gives the same results as the analyses performed at the beginning of this chapter. The concept is extended to include more than one independent variable in the model, so that it is possible to see which factors in combination are associated with the outcome. Data shown in the worked examples in this chapter are from a manual handling occupational study.

THE AIMS OF THIS CHAPTER ARE:

- To revisit probabilities to learn about odds and odds ratios.
- To learn when logistic regression should be used.
- To discover how to do logistic regression using SPSS.
- To interpret the results of logistic regression.

Lower Back pain* Is Your job stressful? Crosstabulation
Count

| | | Is your job stressful? | | Total |
		stress free	stressful	
Lower Back	No LBP	96	44	140
Pain	LBP	34	37	71
Total		130	81	211

FIGURE 12.1   CROSSTABULATION OF LOWER BACK PAIN AND WHETHER THE JOB IS STRESSFUL

PROBABILITY, ODDS AND ODDS RATIOS

Odds and odds ratios are used to express differences in possible explanatory factors (these are called independent variables when this is applied to logistic regression in SPSS later in this chapter) in case–control studies (Chapter 3). This is because relative risks (Chapter 8) would be meaningless, as case–control studies start with a given number of participants who enter the study with and without the disease or condition of interest, so the study design means it is impossible to estimate the risk of developing the disease or condition of interest.

Additionally odds ratios are reported when data are analysed using logistic regression (explained further later in this chapter). Odds ratios can be calculated using two by two tables (crosstabulations) like those used to calculate chi-square statistics shown in Chapter 8. In this example, the dependent variable is Lower Back pain and the independent variable is whether the job is stressful. The resulting crosstabulation is shown in Figure 12.1.

> The probability of having Lower Back pain for a person with a stressful job is: 37/81.
> The probability of not having Lower Back pain, for a person with a stressful job is: 44/81.

These probabilities can be put together to give the odds of having Lower Back pain for a person with a stressful job: (37/81)/(44/81). Using cancelling and manipulating the fractions this simplifies to 37/44 = 0.84. The people in this study are slightly less likely to have Lower Back pain than not.

Similar probabilities can be set up for those without a stressful job giving the odds of having Lower Back pain without a stressful job as: 34/96 = 0.35.

The general scheme of which numbers to use to obtain the probabilities and odds is shown using the diagram shown in Table 12.1. If this is related to the example in Figure 12.1, the disease is Lower Back pain and the possible explanatory factor is a stressful job. 'a' represents those who reported Lower Back pain and a stressful job; 'd' represents those who did not report Lower Back pain nor a stressful job.

TABLE 12.1   SCHEMATIC DIAGRAM OUTLINING A
CROSSTABULATION TO CALCULATE PROBABILITIES, ODDS
AND ODDS RATIOS

	Possible explanatory factor		
	No	Yes	Total
Disease absent	d	c	c+d
Disease present	b	a	a+b
Total	b+d	a+c	a+b+c+d

In general (using the scheme shown in Table 12.1):

The probability of having the disease or condition of interest and the possible explanatory factor is $a/(a+c)$.

The probability of not having the disease or condition of interest, but having the possible explanatory factor is $c/(a+c)$.

The odds of having the disease or condition of interest and the possible explanatory factor is $(a/(a+c))/(c/(a+c))$, which cancels to a/c.

Note: the letters shown in the schematic agree with the ordering in Figure 12.1, and are also in the same order as many other textbooks.

The odds ratio is the quantity usually reported. This is the ratio of the odds of the condition with a given characteristic to the odds of the condition for those without the characteristic. With reference to Table 12.1 this is calculated as $(a/c)/(b/d)$, which can be rearranged to ad/bc. In the Lower Back pain example shown in Figure 12.1, the odds ratio is $(37/44)/(34/96) = (37 \times 96)/(44 \times 34) = 2.37$. In this example $(37/44)$ is the odds of having the condition (Lower Back pain) and the characteristic of interest (stressful job), whilst $(34/96)$ is the odds of having the condition of interest (Lower Back pain) without the given characteristic (stressful job). The odds ratio indicates that those with a stressful job were 2.37 times more likely to have Lower Back pain than those without a stressful job. Note: this is very different from the relative risk for these data calculated in Chapter 8. Relative risks and odds ratios are only similar when the disease, condition or event in question is rare. This is not the case for Lower Back pain as 34% of participants $(71/211)$ in this study suffered from lower back pain (Figure 12.1).

Odds ratios can take any value between 0 and infinity, but not negative values, with the event (dependent variable) in question being more likely to occur if the odds ratio is greater than one and less likely to occur if it is less than one. It is possible to calculate 95% confidence intervals around odds ratios, although these are not easy to calculate by hand and SPSS readily calculates them. In terms of interpretation of 95% confidence intervals for odds ratios, regardless of whether the p-value is present, significance can be assessed by whether the 95% confidence interval includes one (the null value). If the 95% confidence interval does not include one then statistical significance has been achieved. For the Lower Back pain and stressful job example shown in this chapter the 95% confidence interval is 1.321, 4.369, and the p-value is 0.004 using the chi-square test, indicating a significant association between Lower Back pain and having a stressful job.

SPSS calculates odds ratios and 95% confidence intervals for two by two crosstabulations from the crosstab commands. However, use this with care and make sure the

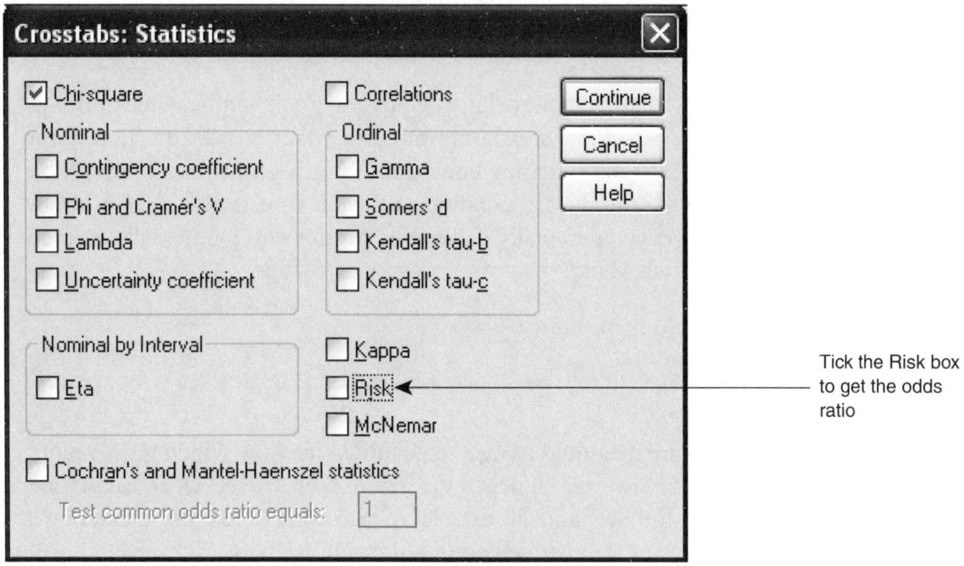

Crosstabs: Statistics

☑ Chi-square   ☐ Correlations   [Continue]

Nominal   Ordinal   [Cancel]
☐ Contingency coefficient   ☐ Gamma
                                              [Help]
☐ Phi and Cramér's V   ☐ Somers' d
☐ Lambda   ☐ Kendall's tau-b
☐ Uncertainty coefficient   ☐ Kendall's tau-c

Nominal by Interval   ☐ Kappa
☐ Eta   ☐ Risk ◄——————— Tick the Risk box to get the odds ratio
           ☐ McNemar

☐ Cochran's and Mantel-Haenszel statistics
    Test common odds ratio equals: [1]

FIGURE 12.2   CROSSTABS: STATISTICS DIALOG BOX

Risk Estimate

	Value	95% Confidence Interval	
		Lower	Upper
Odds Ratio for Lower Back pain (No LBP/LBP)	2.374	1.321	4.269
For cohort Is your job stressful? = stress free	1.432	1.096	1.871
For cohort Is your job stressful? = stressful	.603	.433	.840
N of Valid cases	211		

Use this line to get the odds ratio and 95% confidence interval

Do not use the statistics in these rows

FIGURE 12.3   RISK ESTIMATE OUTPUT FOR THE LOWER BACK PAIN AND STRESSFUL JOB EXAMPLE

coding of the two variables are such that you get the answer expected. To do this, from the Crosstabs dialog box in SPSS (see Chapter 8), click the Statistics button to give the dialog box shown in Figure 12.2. On this dialog box tick Chi-square and Risk, then click Continue to return to the Crosstabs dialog box. Then click OK to give the output; this is shown in Figure 12.3 for the Lower Back pain and stressful job data.

Interpretation

Figure 12.3 shows that having a stressful job was associated with more than a twofold increase in odds of Lower Back pain (OR 2.37; 95% CI 1.32, 4.27).

LOGISTIC REGRESSION

Logistic regression is a statistical modelling technique to investigate relationships between independent variables and a dichotomous dependent variable. Dichotomous means in two categories, so the outcome could be having a given disease, condition or event versus not having the disease, condition or event or pass versus fail a health status test. For example, developmentally delayed versus not developmentally delayed or wheezing versus not wheezing.

Digression to dichotomisation

Some health status tests are measured using a standardised measure which gives a score (a continuous variable). However, clinicians are often keen to see what factors are associated with a poor (or occasionally excellent) performance on the measure, so dichotomise the measure at a standardised point representing a poor (or excellent) performance. These may be a given number of standard deviations below (or above) the standardised mean for that measure. For example, the Bayley Scales of Infant Development (Bayley, 1993) have a standardised mean of 100 and standard deviation of 15, the dichotomisation often occurs at 70, two standard deviations below the mean. Whilst this gives a cut-off for poor performance, a large amount of information is lost by only having two possible outcome states (developmentally delayed versus not developmentally delayed), compared with the full range of scale using the original measure.

It could also be argued that by dichotomising a measure something slightly different to the original scale is being measured. Using the Bayley Scales of Infant Development example, the continuous scale is measuring actual attainment whereas if the cut-off of 70 is being used, developmental delay is being measured.

Back to logistic regression

The independent variables can be categorical or continuous. Results from logistic regression are usually expressed as odds ratios. That is the ratio of the odds of an event for those with a given characteristic to the odds of the event for those without the characteristic. Where the independent variable is continuous, the odds ratios are given for a one unit change. For example, for birthweight measured in kilograms, the odds ratio would be for a one kilogram change in birthweight. Odds are not reported as a result of logistic regression but are useful to show how odds ratios are calculated as shown earlier in this chapter. However, if a unit change greater than one unit (for example 3kg versus 1kg = a two unit change) is required to be reported then the odds ratio needs to be multiplied by itself (squared). For example, if the odds ratio was 1.1 for a one unit change, then for a two unit change it would be $1.1 \times 1.1 = 1.1^2 = 1.21$. This odds ratio would be the same for any two unit change with an odds ratio of 1.1. For a three unit change the odds ratio would be $1.1 \times 1.1 \times 1.1 = 1.1^3 = 1.33$, that is the odds ratio would need to be cubed.

The general null and alternative hypotheses for each variable (separately) included in a logistic regression model is:

H_0: There is no relationship between the dependent variable and the independent variable in question.

H_1: There is a relationship between the dependent variable and the independent variable in question.

Using the Lower Back pain example introduced earlier in this chapter, the specific null and alternative hypotheses are:

H_0: There is no relationship between Lower Back pain and having a stressful job.

H_1: There is a relationship between Lower Back pain and having a stressful job.

Data considerations for doing logistic regression

The dependent variable should be coded 0 and 1, with the category of most importance to the research question taking the coding of 1. For example, using the Lower Back pain dataset already cited in this chapter, absence of Lower Back pain would be coded 0 and presence of Lower Back pain would be coded 1, as the research question would relate to factors associated with Lower Back pain.

Dummy variables for categorical variables do not need to be explicitly constructed for logistic regression as was the case for linear regression (Chapter 11), although some thought should be put into the most appropriate category to be the reference category. This will be explained further later in this chapter.

DOING LOGISTIC REGRESSION USING SPSS

Initially, a series of regressions using one independent variable (in a similar way to simple linear regression in Chapter 11) may be performed. These are sometimes called unadjusted regressions because no other variables are included in the model to modify the effect of the variable in question. To do this in SPSS, click on Analyze → Regression → Binary Logistic… to give the dialog box shown in Figure 12.4. Transfer the dependent variable into the Dependent: box. With this dataset, the presence or absence of Lower Back pain is the dependent variable. Transfer the independent variable(s) to the Covariates: box. As we are going to start simply, only one variable will be added first. To continue with the example from earlier in this chapter the presence or absence of a stressful job will be used.

When a categorical independent variable has been added to the Covariates: box, click on Categorical… to give the dialog box shown in Figure 12.5.

In Figure 12.5, the only variable in the Covariates: box is categorical (stressful job), so should be transferred to the Categorical Covariates: box. The reference category can also be changed. This is the category that is used for comparison. The default is to use the last category (that is the highest coded) as the reference category. However, it is wise to think about which is the best category for the reference category, and if

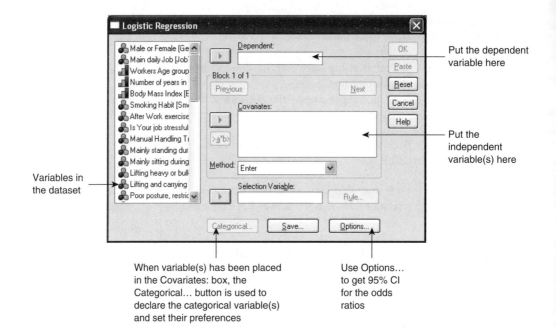

Put the dependent variable here

Put the independent variable(s) here

Variables in the dataset

When variable(s) has been placed in the Covariates: box, the Categorical... button is used to declare the categorical variable(s) and set their preferences

Use Options... to get 95% CI for the odds ratios

FIGURE 12.4   LOGISTIC REGRESSION DIALOG BOX

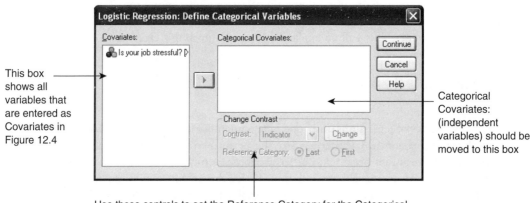

This box shows all variables that are entered as Covariates in Figure 12.4

Categorical Covariates: (independent variables) should be moved to this box

Use these controls to set the Reference Category for the Categorical Covariates (independent variables)

FIGURE 12.5   LOGISTIC REGRESSION: DEFINE CATEGORICAL VARIABLES DIALOG BOX

the desired category is not coded as the first or last (lowest or highest) category, then the variable should be recoded (Chapter 2) so that the category intended as the reference has either the highest or lowest coding.

There may be one category which it would be intuitive to be the reference category; for example, if level of smoking was the independent variable of interest, it would be sensible for non-smokers to be the comparison category. The independent variable may be ethnic group, which in the case of UK data, it is

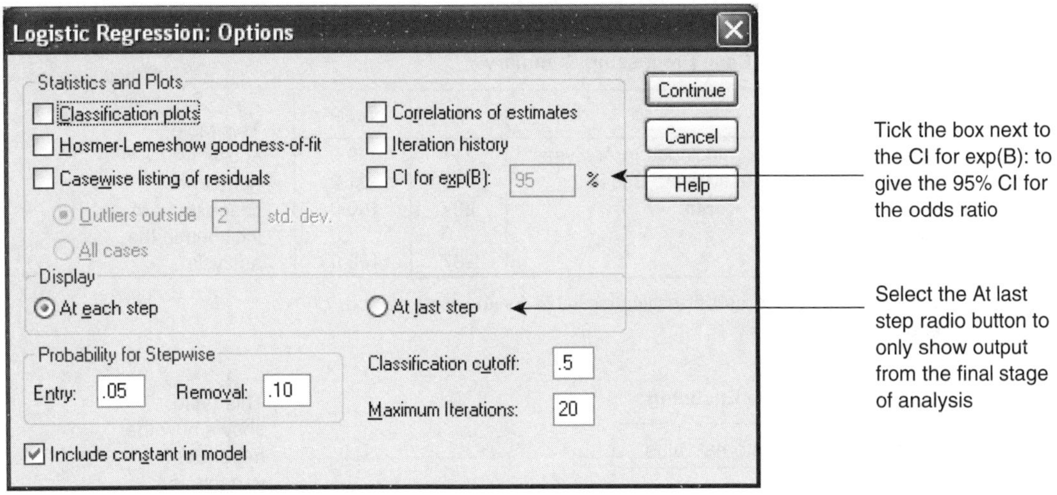

FIGURE 12.6   LOGISTIC REGRESSION: OPTIONS DIALOG BOX

sensible to use 'whites' as the reference group, thus comparing other categories with whites in analysis. If the missing data category is being retained for analysis purposes (occasionally this is the case), it is not sensible to use the missing category as the comparison category because missing data is not likely to have similar characteristics with regard to the variable in question so interpretation may be problematic. A final point worth noting about the choice of reference category is that it is not advisable for the reference category to be one which includes few participants.

To obtain the same result as calculated by hand earlier in this chapter and also using the risk estimate shown in Figure 12.3, the reference category should be the first (in the Lower Back pain example, this is absence of stress at work). When all options related to categorical variables have been selected, click Continue to go back to the Logistic regression dialog box (Figure 12.4). When all options related to categorical variables have been selected, click Continue to go back to the Logistic regression dialog box (Figure 12.4).

Next, click on the Options button to give the Logistic Regression: Options dialog box shown in Figure 12.6. On this dialog box tick CI for exp(B):, leaving the percentage at 95 to give the 95% CI for the odds ratio. The odds ratio is expressed as exp(B) in SPSS because the odds ratios are calculated by antilogging (exponentiating) the beta coefficient (sometimes called the log odds ratio) resulting from modelling. Then click Continue to go back to the Logistic Regression dialog box (Figure 12.4). Then click on OK.

The output from this logistic regression is shown in Figure 12.7. SPSS gives a vast amount of output, much of which is not needed when the results are presented in a report, dissertation, paper or thesis. The main table of interest with the information to be reported is in the final table of the output in Figure 12.7 (entitled Variables in the Equation). Reading across the columns from left to right this table shows the log odds ratio (B), the standard error of the log odds ratio (SE), Wald, degrees of freedom (df), p-value (Sig.), odds ratio (Exp(B)) and 95% CI for the odds ratio (95% CI for Exp(B)). From the final table in Figure 12.7 (and the outputs shown in Figures 12.8 and 12.9); the only statistics that are reported in reports, dissertations, papers or theses are odds ratios, 95% confidence intervals and (sometimes) p-values. For ways to do this see Freeman et al., 2008 or Peacock and Kerry, 2007.

Logistic Regression

Case Processing Summary

Unweighted Cases[a]		N	percent
Selected Cases	Included in Analyses	211	79.0
	Missing Cases	56	21.0
	Total	267	100.0
Unselected Cases		0	.0
Total		267	100.0

This table shows the number of cases that are included in the analysis

[a]If weight is in effect, see classification table for the total number of cases.

Dependent Variable Encoding

Original value	Internal value
No LBP	0
LBP	1

This table shows how the dependent variable is coded

Categorical Variables Codings

		Frequency	Parameter Coding (1)
Is your job stressful?	stress free	130	.000
	stressful	81	1.000

This table shows how the independent variable is coded and the number of participants who gave a positive response to each category.

Block 0: Beginning Block

Classification Table[a, b]

			Predicted		
			Lower Back pain		
			No LBP	LBP	Percentage Correct
	Observed				
Step 0	Lower Back pain	No LBP	140	0	100.0
		LBP	71	0	.0
	Overall Percentage				66.4

[a]Constant is included in the model.
[b]The cut value is .500

Variables in the Equation

		B	S.E.	Wald	df	Sig.	Exp(B)
Step 0	Constant	−.679	.146	21.717	1	.000	.507

The Variables in the Equation table gives the results of modelling without including the independent variable (that is, including the constant only).

(Continued)

FIGURE 12.7   (*Continued*)

Variables not in the Equation

			Score	df	Sig.
Step 0	Variables	Xstress(1)	8.521	1	.004
	Overall Statistics		8.521	1	.004

Xstress is the variable name related to whether the job is stressful or not.

Block 1: Method = Enter

Omnibus Tests of Model Coefficients

		Chi-square	df	Sig.
Step 1	Step	8.428	1	.004
	Block	8.428	1	.004
	Model	8.428	1	.004

Model Summary

Step	−2 Log likelihood	Cox & Snell R Square	Nagelkerke R Square
1	261.096[a]	.039	.054

[a]Estimation terminated at iteration number 4 because parameter estimates changed by less than .001.

Classification Table[a]

			Predicted		
			Lower Back pain		
	Observed		No LBP	LBP	Percentage Correct
Step 1	Lower Back pain	No LBP	140	0	100.0
		LBP	71	0	.0
	Overall Percentage				66.4

[a]The cut value is .500.

Variables in the Equation

		B	S.E.	Wald	df	Sig.	Exp(B)	95.0% C.I. for EXP(B) Lower	Upper
Step 1[a]	Xstress(1)	.865	.299	8.347	1	.004	2.374	1.321	4.269
	Constant	−1.038	.200	27.051	1	.000	.354		

[a]Variable(s) entered on step 1: Xstress.

FIGURE 12.7   OUTPUT FROM THE LOWER BACK PAIN AND STRESSFUL JOB LOGISTIC REGRESSION

Interpretation

Looking at the final table in Figure 12.7, the odds ratio for Lower Back pain with a stressful job compared to those without a stressful job is 2.37 (95% CI 1.32, 4.27). This is highly significant, p-value of 0.004, which is exactly the same as given by the chi–square test.

Including more independent variables

Logistic regression can be extended to include a number of independent variables, which can be a mixture of continuous and categorical variables. However, variables should be chosen systematically. Further variables to be added to logistic regression from this dataset, using Lower Back pain as the dependent variable were selected using chi-square tests (not shown), with those that were significant being included in the modelling process. These were then all added to a logistic regression to give the model shown in Figure 12.8 (previous output in this modelling is suppressed here). Independent variables (variable names given in brackets) entered into the modelling process were gender (Gender), whether the job is stressful (Xstress), the amount of standing the job involves (XStandingjob), the amount of lifting heavy items the job involves (XLifting), the amount of lifting and carrying heavy items the job involves (XLiftingAndCarrying), the degree to which the participant has poor posture and

Variables in the Equation

		B	S.E.	Wald	df	Sig.	Exp(B)	95.0% C.I. for Exp(B) Lower	Upper
Step 1[a]	Gender(1)	−.933	.826	1.278	1	.258	.393	.078	1.984
	Xstress(1)	.896	.320	7.855	1	.005	2.450	1.309	4.585
	XStandingjob			2.285	2	.319			
	XStandingjob(1)	−.193	.441	.192	1	.661	.824	.347	1.957
	XStandingjob(2)	.467	.440	1.126	1	.289	1.595	.673	3.781
	XLifting			.259	2	.879			
	XLifting(1)	.565	1.234	.210	1	.647	1.760	.157	19.771
	XLifting(2)	.557	1.321	.178	1	.673	1.746	.131	23.265
	XLiftingAndCarrying			.059	2	.971			
	XLiftingAndCarrying(1)	−.090	1.231	.005	1	.941	.914	.082	10.196
	XLiftingAndCarrying(2)	.216	1.320	.027	1	.870	1.241	.093	16.489
	XPostureR			1.018	2	.601			
	XPostureR(1)	−.384	.421	.829	1	.363	.681	.298	1.556
	XPostureR(2)	−.075	.440	.029	1	.864	.928	.391	2.198
	Constant	−1.454	.420	11.985	1	.001	.234		

[a]Variable(s) entered on step 1: Gender, Xstress, XStandingjob, XLiftingAndCarrying, XPostureR.

FIGURE 12.8   OUTPUT FROM THE LOWER BACK PAIN MODELLING POSSIBLE EXPLANATORY FACTORS

Variables in the Equation

	B	S.E.	Wald	df	Sig.	Exp(B)	95.0% C.I. for Exp(B)	
							Lower	Upper
Step 1[a] Xstress(1)	.796	.306	6.762	1	.009	2.217	1.217	4.040
XStandingjob			7.875	2	.019			
XStandingjob(1)	−.048	.402	.014	1	.904	.953	.434	2.094
XStandingjob(2)	.854	.346	6.072	1	.014	2.349	1.191	4.632
Constant	−1.311	.275	22.667	1	.000	.270		

[a]Variable(s) entered on step 1: Xstress, XStandingjob.

FIGURE 12.9   FINAL LOWER BACK PAIN MODEL

restricted movement while working (XPostureR). Note: although variables and categories are labelled in the dataset, these are not used in regression output.

In Figure 12.8, where an independent variable has more than two categories, each category (apart from the reference category) has its own p-value; however, for assessing whether a variable is significant overall in the model, the overall significance of the variable needs to be assessed. This is given by SPSS on the line without the number. For example, for the variable XStandingjob there are three rows in Figure 12.8: XStandingjob, XStandingjob(1) and XStandingjob(2). The overall p-value for this variable is shown on the row Xstandingjob and the column Sig. so the overall p-value for this variable is 0.319. If, like for XStandingjob in Figure 12.9 one (or more) category within a variable appears to be non-significant, no attempt should be made to remove that category because the overall significance of the variable is most important. Additionally, if a variable is recoded so that part of it is removed, some participants may be removed from the analysis, which has the potential to change the inferences from modelling.

Sometimes it is sensible to keep non-significant variables in a model to control for their effect (for example, the effect of age or gender). In the example shown in Figure 12.8 it is more sensible to remove non-significant variables (there is no justification to retain gender in this model). However, rather than removing them all at once it is sensible to remove the variable with the largest p-value then refit the model. This is because when one variable is removed from a model, the significance of those left in the model changes. This process is repeated until all variables in the model are significant (with the possible exception of the variables that are being controlled for). The final model using this dataset is shown in Figure 12.9 (intermediate models are not shown).

Interpretation

Figure 12.9 shows that with further modelling, the two variables that remain significantly associated with Lower Back pain are whether the job is stressful and the amount of standing the job involves. It shows that Lower Back pain is 2.22 times more likely in those with a stressful job compared to those without a stressful job (95% CI 1.22, 4.04). Those who stand most of the time in their job are 2.35 times more likely to have Lower Back pain compared to those who do not stand whilst working (95% CI 1.19, 4.63).

SUMMARY

- To execute logistic regression click on Analyze → Regression → Binary Logistic.

EXERCISES

1 Which variables in Figure 12.8 are not statistically significant?

TABLE 12.2   RESULTS OF LOGISTIC REGRESSION TO DETERMINE FACTORS AFFECTING LANGUAGE DELAY IN CHILDREN BORN EXTREMELY PRETERM

Variable	Odds ratio	95% confidence interval
Age at time outcome was measured (years)	0.29	(0.01, 7.92)
Female sex	Reference	
Male sex	1.81	(0.91, 3.61)
Length of hospital stay (days)	1.01	(1.00, 1.02)
Standardised weight at 24 months	0.68	(0.51, 0.91)
No disability	Reference	
Mild disability	1.68	(0.80, 3.52)
Severe disability	9.15	(3.04, 27.56)

Source: Marston et al., 2009

2 In Table 12.2, which factors were not significantly associated with language delay?
3 Why is the 95% confidence interval for length of hospital stay so narrow?
4 Interpret the odds ratios and 95% confidence intervals for level of disability.

APPENDIX 1: DATASETS

The Hotel Employee Diabetes Prevention Awareness and Knowledge Study was a cross-sectional survey in one hotel in the UK asking employees about their knowledge of symptoms and risk factors of diabetes. Questions on current health and lifestyle factors that may influence the probability of getting type 2 diabetes are also asked.

The data for the obesity dataset were collected by students from a convenience sample of their family and friends. Elementary data were collected on diet and exercise as well as respondents' opinions on obesity. In addition, demographic data and anthropometric data were collected, allowing the calculation of body mass index.

The younger women's (age 18 to 49 years) breast awareness survey aimed to discover whether there was a difference in awareness of symptoms and risk factors of breast cancer by age group and ethnicity. Data were collected from students and female employees of a UK university.

The coin tossing exercise used to illustrate probability was carried out in a lecture setting. All students were asked to toss a coin and report the result when prompted to do so. The aim of the experiment was to show students that although there may be a run of one outcome, in the long run it tends towards 50% heads and 50% tails.

The United Kingdom Oscillation Study is a randomised controlled trial of two types of ventilation given to infants born extremely preterm (Johnson et al., 2002). Data were collected from birth to initial hospital discharge then again at 6 months, 12 months and 24 months (Marston et al., 2007; Marston et al., 2009).

The data for the smoking dataset were collected by students from a convenience sample of their family and friends. They asked about smoking status, attitudes and opinions to some smoking related issues and questions on demographics.

The manual handling occupational study aimed to look at workplace factors such as stressful job, posture, frequency of bending and lifting and demographic factors in relation to back pain status in participants.

The dataset on mobility in older people comes from a physiotherapy setting. Data were collected on the falls status of the participants, and then a 'gold standard' test was undertaken by participants to assess their mobility and stability. These data were used to see whether the 'gold standard' test was a good indicator of persistent falls status.

The dataset of participants hospitalised as a result of stroke aims to show there were differences in a number of outcome measures by their discharge destination. The outcome measures were taken at hospital admission, discharge from hospital and five weeks post discharge. Data were also collected on a number of demographic variables which may have been important in explaining these differences.

APPENDIX 2: SOLUTIONS

CHAPTER 1

1 Nominal data, since the responses available are categorical, but unordered.
2 Ordinal data, the possible responses are ordered from never to four or more times a week (when these data are entered into SPSS, never should be coded as the category before once to ensure ordering of the variable; in the questionnaire never appears out of order).
3 Scale data, which is continuous data. The values that respondents could choose are unlimited apart from it being less than or equal to their current age (for consistency). However, it is likely that respondents to this question would report the age they started smoking as their age in years.
4 There were 82 responses to this questionnaire. This can be determined by scrolling down Data View until the final observation is visible. Then look at the grey numbers in the far left of that window to see what is the last one where the data is. The participant ID cannot be used to determine the number of participants in the dataset as sometimes (as with this dataset) these ID numbers do not run consecutively.
5 The variable 'agegroup' is coded such that 1 represents those aged 11 to 30 years, 2 represents 31 to 40 years and 3 representing those aged 41+. These can be shown via the Values column in Variable View (Figure S1).

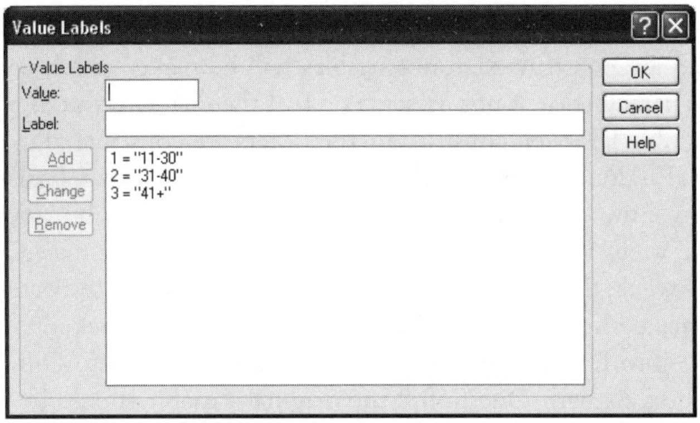

FIGURE S1 VALUE LABELS DIALOG BOX FOR 'AGEGROUP' IN THE OBESITY DATASET

CHAPTER 2

1   To recode a variable, overwriting what is already present, click on Transform →
Recode into Same Variables… . Then put each of the current values in the
Old Value Values box in turn with the corresponding New Value in the Values
box, remembering to click Add between the changes so that they appear in
the Old → New box. When all recodings have been declared click on
Continue then OK. Now go to Variable View to change the Values to reflect
the changes. This is done by clicking on the ▒▒▒ in the relevant Values cell. The
codes and labels can then be changed.

2   To make a new categorical variable from a continuous variable in SPSS,
click on Transform → Recode into Different Variables… to get the Recode
into Different Variables dialog box (Figure S2). BMI should be selected from
the variable list and transferred to the Input Variable → Output Variable:
box. The new variable name should be declared in the Output Variable
Name box and then transferred to the Input Variable → Output Variable:
box using the Change button. Then click on Old and New Values… to
inform SPSS which values should be associated with which category (this
dialog box is shown in Figure S3). It is easiest to deal with the missing data
first selecting the radio button for System- or user-missing from the left of
the dialog box and the System-missing radio button from the right of the
dialog box. Remember to click Add. Then declare those who are obese. The
easiest (and quickest) way to do this is to use the Range, value through
HIGHEST:, where 30 is the value, and the new value for this is 1. Finally, it
is known that if data are not missing or the respondent is not obese then
they must have a BMI less than 30, so on the left of the dialog box use the
All other values radio button, and declare the new code on the right as 0.
Value labels, variable labels, declaring the correct data type and reducing the
number of decimal places can be done in Variable View. The resulting frequencies of this new variable can be seen in Figure S4.

Note: This variable does not have to be coded 0 and 1; it can be coded using any
two distinctive numbers, for example 1 and 2. However, 0 and 1 are beneficial
for regression analysis (shown in later chapters).

3   Figure S5 shows the frequencies for exercise as one variable. When dummy
variables are constructed, four variables will be made, which will be coded 0
(if the characteristic is not present) or 1 (if the characteristic is present). Once
one variable has been constructed, the others are constructed in a similar way.
This is also done using Recode into Different Variables… . First it is necessary
to know how the original variable is coded. This can be ascertained using
Variable View. For exercise they are 0, 1, 2, 3 and 4 for never, once a week,
twice a week, three times a week and 4+ times a week respectively.

   To make the dummy variable for once a week click on Transform →
Recode into Different Variables… to get the Recode into Different Variables
dialog box. As with Question 2 the original variable should be moved to the

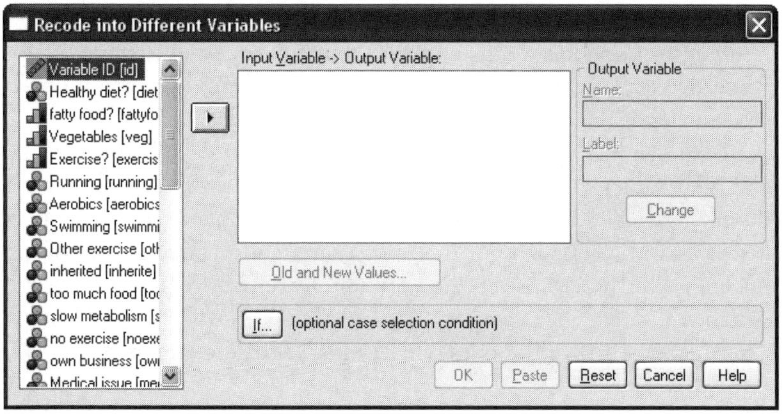

FIGURE S2   RECODE INTO DIFFERENT VARIABLES DIALOG BOX

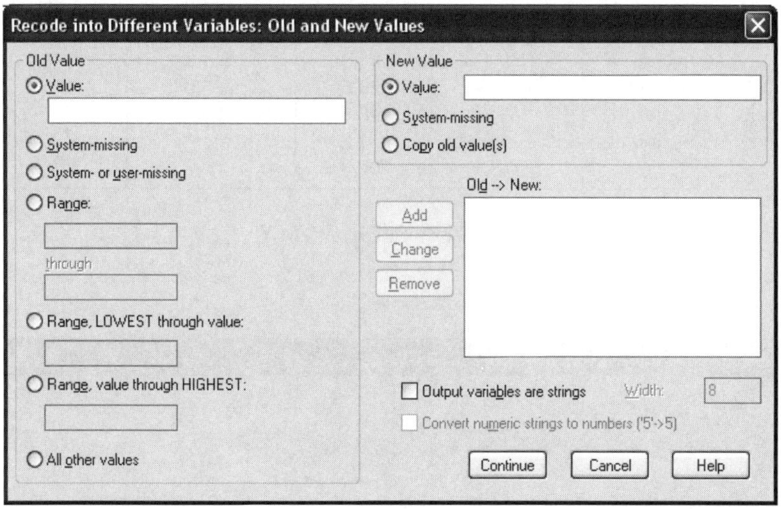

FIGURE S3   RECODE INTO DIFFERENT VARIABLES: OLD AND NEW VALUES DIALOG BOX

obese

		Frequency	Percent	Valid Percent	Cumulative Percent
Valid	not obese	60	73.2	82.2	82.2
	obese	13	15.9	17.8	100.0
	Total	73	89.0	100.0	
Missing	System	9	11.0		
Total		82	100.0		

FIGURE S4   FREQUENCY TABLE SHOWING THE NUMBER AND PERCENTAGE THAT ARE OBESE

Input Variable → Output Variable: box. As four dummy variables are going to result, it is a good idea to give them systematic names, so exercise once a week could be exer1. In addition, as in Question 2 missing data should be considered such that the same participants have missing data in the dummy variables as in the original exercise variable. The Recode into Different Variables: Old and New Values should look like Figure S6 to make the exercise once a week dummy variable. It shows that only those who exercised once a week are coded 1, and all other frequencies of exercise are coded 0 (missing remains missing). This process is repeated for other exercise frequencies except never which is the reference category.

4 The smallest BMI in the obesity dataset is 17.61, the largest BMI is 42.41.

Exercise?

		Frequency	Percent	Valid Percent	Cumulative Percent
Valid	never	27	32.9	33.3	33.3
	1/week	12	14.6	14.8	48.1
	2/week	12	14.6	14.8	63.0
	3/week	9	11.0	11.1	74.1
	4+/week	21	25.6	25.9	100.0
	Total	81	98.8	100.0	
Missing	System	1	1.2		
Total		82	100.0		

FIGURE S5   FREQUENCY TABLE FOR EXERCISE FREQUENCY

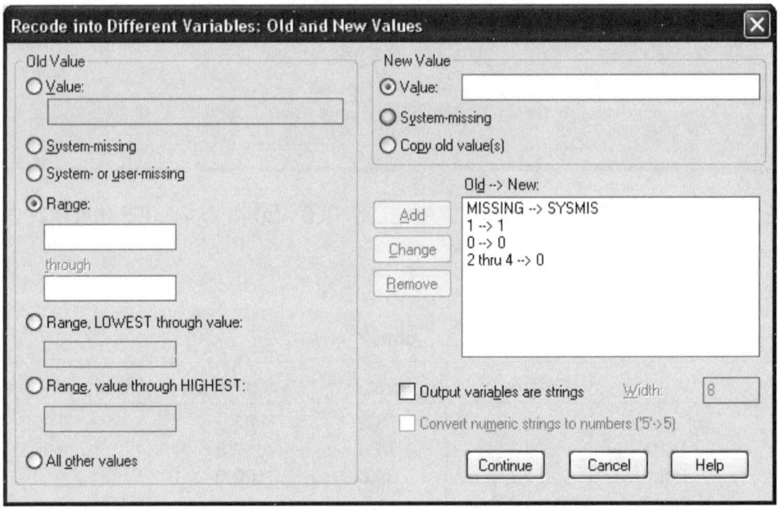

FIGURE S6   RECODE INTO DIFFERENT VARIABLES: OLD AND NEW VALUES DIALOG BOX SHOWING THE RECODING NECESSARY TO MAKE THE DUMMY VARIABLE INDICATING EXERCISE ONCE A WEEK

CHAPTER 3

1   Cases and controls were matched on some baseline variables (age, gender, ethnicity and hospital) to ensure the study population were similar in terms of those factors, and will therefore not need to control for them in statistical analysis.

2   It can be difficult to find matched controls for cases if too many factors are used for matching, which may take a large amount of time and other resources. In addition, if too many factors are used as matching criteria, then there is a risk of overmatching. In doing so factors that may be important in determining a relationship with the outcome may be matched upon meaning that the research may not show the correct results.

3   Controls were selected from the same hospital as the cases so that they could be matched on hospital (a proxy for geographical area), making the participants come from the same population as far as possible. It is also likely that controls were selected from the same hospital as cases for logistical reasons; that is, the study coordinators did not have to visit additional centres to recruit participants. This would have had an impact on the time taken to complete the study, the cost of the study and possibly ethical approval (depending on the rules regarding ethical approval in Spain).

    Controls had different diseases to the cases so that it could be determined as well as possible whether exposures were related to the condition the cases had (bladder cancer in this example).

4   This is a cross sectional study, potential sports people were only assessed once by the Institute of Sports Medicine.

5   With this study the disadvantages of the cross sectional nature of the design is that if someone passes their examination this year there is no guarantee that they are fit to compete next year. Conversely, if someone is unfit to compete today, it might be that they may be fit enough to compete at a later date (depending on the reasons for their assessment failure), but if the system of assessment at the Italian Institute of Sports medicine is truly cross sectional there would be no 'second chance'.

6   This is a randomised controlled trial (RCT).

7   Terms from the extract which lead to this conclusion are a random number sequence being placed into sealed envelopes. This is so that the allocated arm of treatment could not be known in advance. The term arm suggests RCT as this is how the two allocated groups are referred to. The final term from the extract which implies a randomised controlled trial is not blind to allocation. Blinding only occurs in randomised controlled trials. In this RCT it would not be possible to blind the participant or the nurse as it was a smoking cessation trial of usual care versus additional support. The participant would know whether they were receiving additional support and likewise the nurse would have to know which participants were allocated to additional support.

8   If envelopes had been opened, the allocation revealed and either the nurse or the participant had decided that they did not agree with the allocation so

opened another envelope to get the other allocation this introduces bias into the study. A reason for randomising is to balance baseline characteristics; and this is not likely to be the case if participants are effectively selecting their trial arm. This would affect the integrity of the trial as randomised controlled trials are considered to be the 'gold standard' of research studies.

9 The advantage of participants attending their initial appointments together receiving the same allocation is that the possibility of contamination is eliminated: that is, if they were randomised to different arms of the study it is likely that they would share information and therefore it would not be possible to tell whether the outcome was due to their allocation or the one the other person was allocated. Of course, these participants could still encourage one another, but this could equally happen in households where there was only one person involved in the trial.

10 The fact that the question uses the phrase 'over time' suggests that a longitudinal study design is needed – most likely a cohort study. It would not be possible or ethical to carry out a randomised controlled trial with assessments over time because it is not likely to be possible to randomise participants to a given lifestyle as some lifestyles are known to be harmful (such as smoking, excessive alcohol consumption or a diet high in fat, salt and/or sugar). To assess the impact on health it may be necessary to study this cohort over a long period of time (depending on the outcome). The outcome is likely to be the onset of a given condition such as CHD or death from a specific condition related to lifestyle.

Next comes the question of where to obtain participants from, and which population they are representing. If the aim of the study is to represent the country the study is being carried out in, then a random sample of the population in question would be needed. However, this is rarely practical, so either all persons or a random sample of persons from a specific place may be used (with the caveat that the results are representing that population, which could be a smaller geographical population or an occupational population). If it was to be an occupational cohort, participants could be recruited by approaching the employer(s) and allowing access to their employees. Recruitment and retention may also be good because a number of employees are taking part in the study. It may also be possible to do some assessments in the workplace, which would also minimise the inconvenience to participants. Other aspects of inclusion that may need to be thought about include age. If the outcome is a condition that is not usually seen until later life, unless money is no object, it would not make sense to follow participants from their teens (or possibly not twenties either).

Then there is the question of how to assess the participants that should be considered. Physical measurements to assess factors such as weight, height, waist and hip measurements, blood pressure and blood lipids will be required periodically. These will be expensive to carry out if they are done by the study team as it is necessary to meet all participants to collect these data. Other data (such as information on diet, smoking, alcohol consumption and exercise) may be collected via questionnaires. Where possible these should be validated questionnaires. These are cheaper to administer than physical examinations so information may be sought this way more often than physical examinations (depending on the budget). It is also necessary to think about how the outcomes are going to be reported. Some outcomes could be self-reported (although it may be necessary to have a mechanism that outcomes can be reported between the scheduled data collection times. If death is an outcome thought needs to be put into how these data are collected, as clearly it cannot be self-reported.

CHAPTER 4

1   This question is solved by dividing the number who died from diseases of the circulatory system (88292) by the total number who died (243324). The proportion of males dying of a disease of the circulatory system in 2005 (excluding external factors) was 88292/243324 = 0.363 (36%). This means, of those males who died in 2005, the estimated probability that it was from a disease of the circulatory system was 36%.

2   To solve this question the first thing that must be done is to add the two reported numbers of conceptions to give a total number of conceptions to women in their 20s. Then divide this by the total number of conceptions to discover the proportion of women conceiving in their 20s in 2005. These are: (185500+211300)/841800 = 396800/841800 = 0.471 (47%). The probability of a conception being to a woman in her 20s in 2005 was 47%.

3   This percentage is likely to be inaccurate because of the level of information the Government provides to calculate these percentages. The numbers of conceptions were only reported to the nearest thousand, so it is impossible to tell whether there is under or over reporting of conceptions. Additionally, there will be some conceptions that will be unreported because the foetus is lost before the woman has visited her GP to confirm the pregnancy and register for ante-natal services.

4   The probability of giving birth to a male followed by a female (assuming no external influencing factors) is the probability of giving birth to a male in 2006 multiplied by the probability of having a female. The probability of giving birth to a male was 342429/669601. The probability of having a female can be calculated from the data given since if a woman did not have a male she must have had a female. Therefore, the number of females born was 669601−342429 = 327172. The probability of having a female was 327172/669601.

Having a male followed by a female are independent events, meaning that the outcome of the first event does not influence the outcome of the second event. Therefore the probability of having a male followed by a female is:

$$\frac{342429}{669601} \times \frac{327172}{669601} = 0.51 \times 0.49 = 0.25$$

The probability of a woman having a male followed by a female is 0.25 (25%).

CHAPTER 5

1 For birthweight it is impossible to say what the shape of the distribution is since, whilst the standard deviation is much less than half the mean, this can occur with skewed data too. The standard deviation for number of days to surgery is greater than the mean, so mean $-$ ($2 \times$ SD) would give a negative value which is not possible for number of days to surgery, therefore the data are right skewed.

2 The stem-and-leaf plot shows most men had a BMI between 20kg/m^2 and 24kg/m^2. There were two men with a BMI of 19kg/m^2 and four men with a BMI of 30kg/m^2 or more.

CHAPTER 6

1 Table 6.1 has been redrawn with the numbers and percentages when the missing data have been excluded (Table S1). First, the total number with data present has to be calculated. This is done by taking the total number (N) as it was presented in Table 6.1 and subtracting the number whose data were unknown (= missing) on that variable. For example, for age group, the total number shown in Table 6.1 is 2495. However, there were 96 participants who had missing data, so these have to be subtracted to give the total number with data present: 2495–96 = 2399. Then the new percentages can be calculated. For example, for age 0–19 divide 178 by 2399 to give the proportion of participants who were aged 0–19, then multiply by 100 to give the percentage aged 0–19 (7.4%).

2 Valid percent (the percentage excluding missing data) should be used in preference to percentages that include missing data because participants with missing data add nothing to the analysis, that is, their characteristics are unknown and as such are likely to be a diverse group on whatever variable is selected.

3 Table 6.1 could be further improved by only including one category of the dichotomous variables since it is obvious what the other category is and the numbers and percentages attributed to that category could be calculated. However, this may be considered a matter of taste/style.

4 Fifty-three participants gave a valid response to smoking status (Figure S7). There were no missing data for this variable.

5 Twenty-four participants (45.3%) were never smokers.

6 39.1% of participants thought smokers' breaks were the same length as those of non-smokers (Figure S8). This variable has missing data so it is important that the results in the Valid Percent column are used.

7 It is possible that the missing data are because participants did not have an opinion as to the length of smokers' breaks. This could have been verified by including a 'don't know' option. However, if this was the case, those who responded 'don't know' may be excluded from analysis because participants

TABLE S1   PERCENTAGES AND VALID PERCENTAGES

Variable	With missing data		Without missing data	
	%	n/N	%	n/N
Age				
0–19	7.1	178/2495	7.4	178/2399
20–34	39.0	972/2495	40.5	972/2399
35–59	32.5	812/2495	33.8	812/2399
60+	17.6	437/2495	18.2	437/2399
Unknown	3.9	96/2495		
Sex				
Male	57.4	1433/2495	58.9	1433/2434
Female	40.1	1001/2495	41.1	1001/2434
Unknown	2.4	61/2495		
Birth in UK				
UK born	14.0	273/1951	19.6	273/1390
Not UK born	57.3	1117/1951	80.4	1117/1390
Unknown	28.8	561/1951		
Ethnic origin				
White	17.9	348/1947	22.6	348/1540
Indian sub-continent	22.1	431/1947	28.0	431/1540
Black Caribbean	2.9	56/1947	3.6	56/1540
Black African	25.2	490/1947	31.8	490/1540
Black other	1.7	33/1947	2.1	33/1540
Other	9.4	182/1947	11.8	182/1540
Unknown	20.9	407/1947		

Source: Maguire et al., 2002

Smoking status

		Frequency	Percent	Valid Percent	Cumulative Percent
Valid	Current smoker	13	24.5	24.5	24.5
	Ex-smoker	16	30.2	30.2	54.7
	Never smoker	24	45.3	45.3	100.0
	Total	53	100.0	100.0	

FIGURE S7   SPSS OUTPUT FOR SMOKING STATUS

In relation to non-smokers, are smokers' breaks...?

		Frequency	Percent	Valid Percent	Cumulative Percent
Valid	shorter	4	7.5	8.7	8.7
	the same	18	34.0	39.1	47.8
	longer	24	45.3	52.2	100.0
	Total	46	86.8	100.0	
Missing	9	7	13.2		
Total		53	100.0		

FIGURE S8   SPSS OUTPUT FOR PERCEIVED LENGTH OF SMOKERS' BREAKS

would not have added anything apart from showing explicitly that they do not have an opinion on that question. A disadvantage of including a 'don't know' category is that if there is one on the questionnaire, participants are likely to use it, which could be problematic because there is likely to be more potentially unusable data than would be desirable.

CHAPTER 7

1   The sampling has been done by stratifying by age, such that the percentage in each age group reflects the percentage of people in the workplace in that age group.

2   If I were to carry out the study I would reconsider the oldest age group. This study was carried out in the UK where the retirement age is 65, and whilst there are clearly some people who are continuing to work beyond their 65th birthday, people in the 65 to 75 years age group are likely to be closer to 65 than 75. Therefore, to be inclusive I would have included everyone aged 55+ in the oldest age group (thus only having three age groups). This would have still been statistically significant (p = 0.027) indicating there is a difference in the percentage of people doing piecework by age group.

3   The random element of this study came from the half days which physicians recruited to the study. This is not a random sample of potential participants because they (that is, those working in the area of France where the study was being carried out) did not have an equal probability of being in the sample selected. Although the methods section of the paper says that the physicians were unable to select the study participants, it would have been possible since on the recruiting half days, study participants were always the tenth person to have their annual health check. That means that it would have been possible to know which appointment would give the tenth attendee, so the receptionist (or whoever books the appointments) would potentially be able to give the study appointment (or not give the appointment) to a specific person.

4   It is likely that this study design was chosen for ease of data collection, partly in terms of time and money. Potential participants did not have to visit the physician more than they would anyway (for their annual appointment) and the physicians were working at their normal times in their normal places of work.

5   A way to make the participants of the study randomly selected within physician would have been to take a random sample of potential participants who were registered with each physician, then invite these people to participate in the study.

6   The difference in the mean number of words vocalised is 51−33 = 18.

7   The 95% CI indicates that we can be 95% certain that the mean difference (female−male) in number of words vocalised could be as small as 11.4 words or as large as 24.2 words. This 95% CI does not include 0 (the null value which indicates no difference) so there is good evidence of a real difference in the population from which the sample was drawn.

CHAPTER 8

1   To ensure the null hypothesis is two–sided the one given in the paper by De Tychey et al. (2008) should be altered to: There is no difference in PND level between women who had a male or female infant.
2   The corresponding alternative hypothesis would be: There is a difference in PND level between women who had a male or female infant.

In relation to non-smokers, are smokers' breaks...? × Smoking status Crosstabulation

			Smoking status			
			Current smoker	Ex-smoker	Never smoker	Total
In relation to non-smokers, are smokers' breaks...?	shorter	Count	2	1	1	4
		% within In relation to non-smokers, are smokers' breaks...?	50.0%	25.0%	25.0%	100.0%
		% within Smoking status	20.0%	6.3%	5.0%	8.7%
	the same	Count	7	4	7	18
		% within relation to non-smokers, are smokers' breaks...?	38.9%	22.2%	38.9%	100.0%
		% within Smoking status	70.0%	25.0%	35.0%	39.1%
	longer	Count	1	11	12	24
		% within relation to non-smokers, are smokers' breaks...?	4.2%	45.8%	50.0%	100.0%
		% within Smoking status	10.0%	68.8%	60.0%	52.2%
Total		Count	10	16	20	46
		% within In relation to non-smokers, are smokers' breaks...?	21.7%	34.8%	43.5%	100.0%
		% within Smoking status	100.0%	100.0%	100.0%	100.0%

FIGURE S9   SPSS OUTPUT SHOWING A CROSSTABULATION OF SMOKING STATUS AND PERCEIVED LENGTH OF SMOKERS' BREAKS

Chi-Square Tests

	Value	df	Asymp. Sig. (2-sided)	Exact Sig. (2-sided)	Exact Sig. (1-sided)	Point Probability
Pearson Chi-Square	9.719[a]	4	.045	.041		
Likelihood Ratio	10.681	4	.030	.041		
Fisher's Exact Test	10.013			.023		
Linear-by-Linear Association	4.905[b]	1	.027	.029	.019	.010
N of Valid Cases	46					

[a]4 cells (44.4%) have expected count less than 5. The minimum expected count is 87.
[b]The standardised statistic is 2.215.

FIGURE S10   SPSS OUTPUT OF STATISTICAL TESTS ASSOCIATED WITH SMOKING STATUS AND PERCEIVED LENGTH OF SMOKERS' BREAKS

3   One current smoker thought smokers' breaks are longer than non-smokers breaks (Figure S9).

4   Fisher's exact test was used to determine whether there was a relationship between smoking status and perceived length of smokers' breaks. This was used because more than 20% of cells had an expected count of less than 5 (as shown in footnote 'a' of the Chi-Square Tests table in Figure S10). This means the Chi-Square test is not valid.

5   There was a significant relationship between smoking status and perceived length of smokers' breaks p = 0.023. From the crosstabulation it can be seen that a lower percentage of current smokers than ex-smokers and never smokers perceive smokers' breaks to be longer than non-smokers' breaks. Conversely, a greater percentage of current smokers consider smokers' breaks to be shorter than those of non-smokers.

6   Sensitivity is the proportion of true positives that are also test positive. In the context of this example, it is the proportion that scored below the cut-off on the specified parent reported development index (the test status) and therefore indicate developmental delay of those who scored < 70 on the Bayley MDI (the true status).

7   There is a slight advantage of selecting the parent report composite as the test to determine developmental delay because the sensitivity and specificity are both the highest of those listed. This means there are the fewest false negatives and false positives, meaning that the fewest parents and children are inconvenienced with additional tests if they were false positives and the fewest with developmental delay are missed. Additionally, looking at the construction of the parent report composite (in the explanatory text above the question) shows that it is constructed from non-verbal cognition items as well as vocabulary and sentence complexity, so does not rely totally on one domain (although it is dominated by vocabulary), making it more rounded than the other parent reported measures.

8   The women who agreed on their groupings at both time points were those who were classified in ≤ 11 at both time points or 12–13 at both time points or ≥ 14 at both time points. The total number who agreed was: 122+386+177 = 685 (65% of women).

9 A kappa value of 0.43 indicates moderate agreement.

10 Looking at the data shown in Table 8.2 it is clear that more than a third of women who were questioned about their age at menarche when in middle age could not remember, even when data were categorised. Therefore it may not be worthwhile collecting such data from middle aged women unless it is possible to anchor their age at menarche to other significant life events.

CHAPTER 9

1 The paired t-test was used to analyse the data shown. A number of pairwise comparisons were conducted between time points during and after pregnancy. Data were collected longitudinally so measurements were taken on the same women over time.

2 From the data given, it can be concluded that depression was significantly worse in pregnancy (regardless of the point at which the measurement was taken) than in the postpartum period. However, the mean differences in scores between the two time points were not great, and such small differences may not be clinically significant.

3 It would have been more correct to analyse these data using a repeated measures ANOVA since what is currently presented may be described as multiple testing. Repeated measures ANOVA should be done to test for overall significance and then if necessary post hoc tests done to discover where the differences (if any) were.

4 Figure S11 shows that the mean weight for those who did not exercise in this dataset was 72kg (SD 14kg) and the mean weight for those who exercised was 76kg (SD 14kg). There is not a statistically significant difference in weight by exercise status (p = 0.241), with those who exercise being 4.1kg heavier than those who did not exercise on average (95% CI for the difference −2.8kg, 11.0kg).

5 A causal relationship between weight and exercise status cannot be implied from the results shown in Question 4. The result is not statistically significant. In addition, there are a number of other factors which should be taken into account when considering weight and exercise status such as sex (it was shown in Chapter 9 that there was a significant difference in weight between males and females using the same dataset). Age, diet and other lifestyle factors may also influence weight. Additionally, it is not known whether higher weight came before exercise in this study as the study was cross sectional and asked about current weight and exercise status.

Group Statistics

	any exercise	N	Mean	Std. Deviation	Std. Error Mean
Weight	no	24	71.92	13.622	2.781
	yes	52	76.04	14.354	1.991

(Continued)

FIGURE S11 (*Continued*)

Independent Samples Test

		Levene's Test for Equality of Variances		t-test for Equality of Means						
									95% Confidence Interval of the Difference	
		F	Sig.	t	df	Sig. (2-tailed)	Mean Difference	Std. Error Difference	Lower	Upper
Weight	Equal variances assumed	.032	.858	−1.182	74	.241	−4.122	3.487	−11.070	−2.826
	Equal variances not assumed			−1.205	47.043	.234	−4.122	3.420	−11.001	−2.757

FIGURE S11   INDEPENDENT SAMPLES T-TEST OUTPUT FOR THE ANALYSIS OF WEIGHT BY EXERCISE STATUS

CHAPTER 10

1   The Mann-Whitney U test was used to discover whether there were statistically significant differences between community and conventional therapy. This test was used because there are two separate groups (those randomised to community therapy and those randomised to conventional therapy). In addition, the summary statistics show that the variables are skewed. This can be seen by examining the median in relation to the range. The median shows the value of the middle observation and the range shows the values of the highest and lowest observations, so if the median is closer to the minimum or maximum then the variable will be skewed. For example, in five-metre timed walk the median number of seconds to complete this task in those randomised to community therapy was 10, with a range of 6 to 40 seconds. This means that 50% of participants took 6, 7, 8, 9 or 10 seconds to complete this task. This means this variable was right skewed: with a large amount of data at the lower end of the range, with fewer large values.

2   The median time to complete the five-metre timed walk for those randomised to community therapy was 10 seconds (range 6, 40), compared to 9 seconds (range 6, 70) in those randomised to conventional therapy. This was not statistically significant (p = 0.34).

3   Looking at the outcome measures presented, none of them is statistically significant, indicating that community therapy is no better than conventional treatment. Therefore, it is unlikely that community therapy would be implemented in its current format.

4 This study was analysed using the Mann-Whitney U test.

5 In the usual care group, the median change in outcome between baseline and the end of study was positive (indicating an improvement in their condition); however, the minimum was negative (−2.6), meaning that at least one participant became worse at completing the outcome measure between baseline and the end of the study. This may indicate a worsening of their hand movement over time.

6 Using the rules regarding p-values, 0.06 is considered to be not significant. However, a p-value of 0.06 is approaching significance, so emphasis should be put on the difference in medians with a statement indicating the median difference approached significance with a greater median difference in the origami group.

7 It can be seen from Figure S12 and Figure S13 that all males started smoking between the ages of 10 and 20 years old, whereas females started smoking over a greater range of ages with one participant starting smoking at age 22 and another at 41 years.

The most appropriate statistical test to use is the Mann-Whitney U test because the data comprise a dichotomous variable (sex) and a continuous variable (age at which participants started smoking). The data look fairly Normally distributed with the exception of the outlier seen in the histogram relating to females. Under normal circumstances it would be beneficial to return to the original questionnaire to discover whether this was a data entry error; but this has been done already as I entered the data. It is difficult to know whether the distribution of ages in the population would be Normal (which would be justification for using the independent samples t-test); however, it is likely that there would be a spike at age 16 (the legal age for buying tobacco before 1st October 2007, therefore the socially acceptable answer). In addition, as this is a small dataset (9 males and 16 females) it is better to use a non-parametric test.

The results of the test shown in Figure S14 show that the p-value for this test is approaching significance at $p = 0.074$; so the null hypothesis is accepted. Looking at the table of ranks it can be seen that the mean rank for females is higher than the mean rank for males, indicating an older age at which they started smoking.

8 The boxplot shown in Figure S15 shows that median age at starting smoking was similar for those currently aged up to 34 years and those aged 35 to 44 years. The range of ages that participants were when they started smoking is greatest in those currently aged 35 to 44 years. Median age at commencing smoking was a little lower in those currently aged 45 or older. There was also an outlier in this age group (participant number 26) who commenced smoking in their 40s.

To determine whether there is an association between current age and the age participants started smoking, the Kruskal-Wallis H test was used because there are more than two groups and a continuous variable which was not Normally distributed. The results (shown in Figure S16) show that there was not a significant difference between the groups ($p = 0.204$).

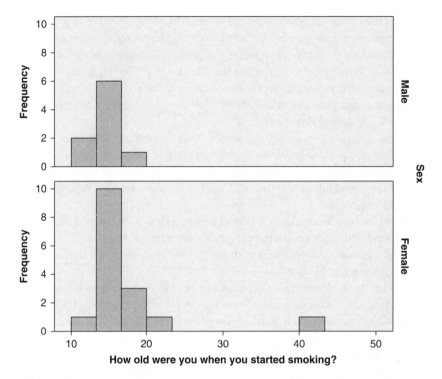

FIGURE S12   HISTOGRAM OF AGE AT WHICH PARTICIPANTS STARTED SMOKING BY SEX

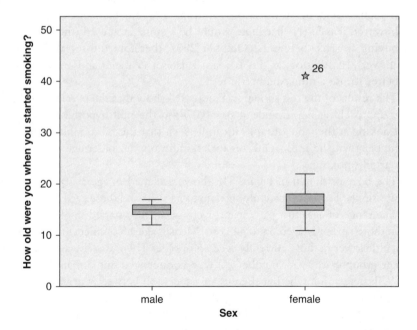

FIGURE S13   BOXPLOTS OF AGE AT WHICH PARTICIPANTS STARTED SMOKING BY SEX

Ranks

	sex	N	Mean Rank	Sum of Ranks
How old were you when you started smoking?	male	9	9.56	86.00
	female	16	14.94	239.00
	Total	25		

Test Statistics[b]

	How old were you when you started smoking?
Mann-Whitney U	41.000
Wilcoxon W	86.000
Z	−1.789
Asymp. Sig. (2-tailed)	.074
Exact Sig. [2*(1-tailed Sig.)]	.084[a]

[a]Not corrected for ties.
[b]Grouping Variable: sex.

FIGURE S14   OUTPUT FROM MANN-WHITNEY U TEST BETWEEN SEX AND AGE AT WHICH PARTICIPANTS STARTED SMOKING

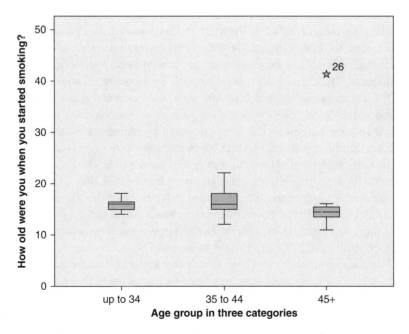

FIGURE S15   BOXPLOTS OF AGE AT STARTING TO SMOKE BY CURRENT AGE GROUP

Ranks

	Age group in	N	Mean Rank
How old were you when you started smoking?	up to 34	11	14.68
	35 to 44	6	14.92
	45+	8	9.25
	Total	25	

Test Statistics[a, b]

	How old were you when you started smoking?
Chi-Square	3.179
df	2
Asymp. Sig.	.204

[a]Kruskal Wallis Test.
[b]Grouping Variable: Age group in three categories.

FIGURE S16 RESULTS OF THE KRUSKAL-WALLIS H TEST FOR AT STARTING TO SMOKE BY CURRENT AGE GROUP

CHAPTER 11

1   The Pearson's correlation coefficient for MDI and linguistic skills is 0.66.
2   The correlation coefficient for MDI and linguistic skills is positive, so as MDI increases, so do linguistic skills. This is expected as they are both developmental outcomes so it is expected that they would both be low in the same participants. The correlation is considered to be moderate to strong.
3   The correlations between linguistic skills and vocabulary and linguistic skills and sentence complexity were so high because the variables were subsets of one another. Linguistic skills were calculated by adding the vocabulary and sentence complexity scores together. Therefore these three variables are measuring the same thing, and no conclusions can be drawn from these correlations.
4   $p < 0.001$ in relation to correlations indicates that the linear correlation observed is significantly different from 0. Remember that the null hypothesis for Pearson's correlation is: there is no linear relationship between the two continuous variables of interest in the population. This equates to the true population correlation coefficient being zero.
5   The correlation coefficient is so low despite the statistical significance being so high because there are a large number of participants in the study (500). With increasing numbers of participants the correlation needed to attain statistical significance decreases rapidly. Where there are 500 participants in a study a Pearson's correlation coefficient of 0.09 will be statistically significant at the 5% level and a Pearson's correlation coefficient of 0.12 will be statistically significant at the 1% level (Bland, 2000).

6   If they had not been significant, the model may have included age at which the dependent variable was measured because it is clear that those who are older are likely to be able to vocalise more words than younger children. Additionally, sex may have been included as there is much evidence in the literature that many outcomes differ by sex, and child development is no exception to that. This analysis bears that out with both variables being statistically significant in the expected directions; number of words vocalised being lower in males and greater with increasing age.

7   In Table 11.3 sex and level of disability are categorical variables. This is made clear in the Table as one category does not have a coefficient associated with it; instead it is shown as the reference category, the one that the other category(ies) are compared to.

8   On average, males vocalised 10.01 fewer words (95% CI −16.08, −3.94) than females, controlling for other variables presented in Table 11.3. The number of words vocalised decreases by 0.16 words (95% CI −0.26, −0.06) for each day spent in hospital in the neonatal period, controlling for the other variables in the model (those shown in Table 11.3). Both variables were statistically significant★. Sex differences in child development had been well documented, with males faring worse in many outcomes. Number of days spent in hospital following birth was an indicator of neonatal illness with those who were sickest spending most time in hospital before initial discharge.

★Statistical significance is indicated by the fact that the 95% confidence intervals do not include zero.

CHAPTER 12

1   The variables that were not significant in Figure 12.8 were: gender, the amount of standing the job involves (XStandingjob), the amount of lifting heavy items the job involves (Xlifting), the amount of lifting and carrying heavy items the job involves (XLiftingAndCarrying) and the degree to which the participant has poor posture and restricted movement while working (XPostureR).

2   Age at which the measure was administered and sex of the child were not significantly associated with language delay. However, it was decided a priori to include these factors in the model because the literature suggests age and sex are strong determinants of language delay. The individual coefficient for mild disability was not statistically significant (the 95% CI straddled 1, the null value for odds ratios); however, the overall variable was significant.

3   The 95% confidence interval for length of hospital stay is so narrow because this is a continuous variable which has a lot of power, and the odds ratio presented represents that for an increase in hospital stay of one day.

4   Those with severe disability were more than nine times more likely to have language delay than those with no disability (OR 9.15, 95% CI 3.04, 27.56) controlling for the other variables in the model (the other variables are shown in Table 12.2).

GLOSSARY

95%: The percentage used in most confidence intervals. Used because it corresponds to statistical significance at the 5% level.

Alternative hypothesis (H_1 or H_A): Hypothesis of difference set up with the null hypothesis before a significance test is carried out. It takes the general form: there is a difference in the population from which the sample is drawn between the two groups on the variable being tested. This can be one sided or two sided depending on how the test is set up.

Association: Two variables are associated with one another if the level of one differs with the level of the other.

Average: A general term referring to a central tendency statistic. When people refer to average they generally mean the 'mean'.

Bar charts: A graph to show the frequency of nominal data.

Binary variable: See dichotomous variable.

Blinding: Concealing the randomised allocation from the participant and/or trial coordinators. Where either the participant or the trial coordinators are aware of the allocation, the trial is single blind. Where neither participant nor trial coordinators are aware of the allocation the trial is double blind.

Boxplot: A graph used for ordinal data, often used to show data by a categorical variable. The graph shows the median (horizontal line within the box), upper and lower quartiles (the horizontal borders of the boxes) and outliers.

Case-control study: This takes a group of people with a disease or condition of interest (the cases) and a group without the disease or condition of interest (the controls). The design is usually retrospective, relating past exposure to possible causal factors to current disease to determine differences between the two groups.

Categorical variable: Data where individuals fall into groups. For example, sex – male/female; smoker/non-smoker; underweight/ideal weight/obese/morbidly obese.

Cell: An individual position in a given row and column in a crosstabulation.

Census: Data collected from the whole population.

Central tendency: The umbrella term used to describe measures to describe the centre of a distribution such as mean and median.

Chi-square test χ^2:   A statistical test used to investigate the relationship between two categorical variables. It is a significance test only (only gives a p-value). Assumptions: used for large samples where at least 80% of the table's cells have expected frequencies greater than five and all cells have expected frequencies greater than one.

Cluster randomised trial: An experimental/interventional study design whereby groups of participants are randomly assigned to treatment groups. For example, GP practices may be randomised so that all participants attending the same GP practice are randomised to the same treatment group. This minimises the possibility of the effect being diluted (if participants find out about the alternative treatment and prefer to be on that). This dilution is especially likely to occur for health promotion interventions such as weight control or smoking cessation trials.

Cluster sampling: Sampling where groups of individuals are selected rather than individuals.

Cohen's Kappa (κ):   Used to measure inter rater agreement to classify observations into a given number of groups. It gives a measure of agreement in excess of that which would happen by chance. Kappa is expressed as a number between 0 and 1 whereby 0 is no agreement and 1 is perfect agreement.

Cohort study: Cohort studies are observational studies used to determine/investigate risk factors for a disease or condition of interest. Participants are usually followed over time (prospectively) to see if they experience the event/disease of interest.

Confidence interval: A measure of how precise an estimate is.

Constant: See intercept.

Contingency table: See crosstabulation.

Continuous data: Data that can take any value within a given range depending on the accuracy of the equipment used for measurement. For example, height, weight.

Crossover trial: A randomised controlled trial where each participant is used as their own control.

Cross sectional study: A single group of subjects is studied at one point in time.

Crosstabulation: A table of two categorical variables to show the numbers and percentages who have given characteristics.

Cumulative frequency: For a given value, it is the number of observations less than or equal to the given value.

Cumulative percentage: The percentage of observations less than or equal to the given value.

Degrees of freedom: Statistical concept, usually an integer, which indicates the number of independent (unrelated) components in a set of data.

Denominator: Total number with valid data for a given variable.

Dependent variable: The variable that is being predicted in regression analysis. The y variable.

Descriptive statistics: Statistics that describe characteristics of the participants in a dataset.

DF: See degrees of freedom.

Dichotomisation: Converting a continuous measure to a categorical one to provide a cut off.

Dichotomous variable: A categorical variable that has two categories. For example sex (male or female), vital status (dead or alive).

Discrete data: Data that can only take a limited number of values, usually integers (whole numbers). For example, number of students in a room, number of deaths in a hospital in a year.

Dispersion: A general term for the spread of the data. This can be measured specifically using the standard deviation, variance, range, minimum, maximum, lower quartile, upper quartile, interquartile range.

Dummy variable: Categorical variables cannot be used in regression analyses in the same way as continuous variables, so with variables that have more than two categories a series of dichotomous variables have to be constructed – these are called dummy variables.

Explanatory variable(s):   See independent variable(s).

Extrapolate: To estimate (a value of a variable outside a known range) from values within a known range by assuming that the estimated value follows logically from the known values. It can be dangerous as impossible values may result.

Fisher's exact test: A significance test to investigate the relationship between two categorical variables. It makes no assumptions about the size of groups, so can be used if data violates the assumptions of the chi-square test.

Frequency: The number of times a given value occurs within a given variable.

Frequency distribution: Set of all possible frequencies for a given variable.

Friedman's test: An extension to the Wilcoxon matched pairs test for three or more time periods.

Gradient: See slope.

Histogram: Used for displaying a frequency distribution for a continuous variable. The x axis (horizontal) shows continuous data. The y axis (vertical) shows the frequency or percentage of the data in a given category.

Hypothesis: An hypothesis is an untested statement. A statement of proposition to be tested in research.

Independent event: Events are independent if knowing the outcome of one event, does not tell us about the outcome of other events.

Independent samples t-test: A significance test which compares the mean of a continuous variable between two groups, for example, the mean height of boys and girls aged two who were born extremely preterm. Assumptions: The variable of interest must be Normally distributed and the variances of the two groups should be equal. It is sometimes referred to as the unpaired t-test or two samples t-test.

Independent variable(s):   The variable(s) that is thought to affect the outcome in regression analysis.

Indicator variable: See dummy variable.

Integer: A positive or negative whole number.

Intention to treat: In randomised controlled trials, data are analysed according to the original randomisation regardless of whether participants swap treatments, drop out or refuse treatments.

Interaction: The modification of the effect of one factor on the outcome by the presence of another factor in the model.

Intercept: In regression, the value of y when x=0.

Kruskal Wallis H test: An extension to the Mann Whitney U test used when there are three or more groups. It is a non-parametric test that provides a p-value only.

Left skew: See negatively skewed.

Logistic regression: A type of regression used when the outcome is dichotomous, for example dead versus alive or diseased versus well.

Longitudinal study: See cohort study.

Mann Whitney U test: A non-parametric test, based on ranks, analogous to the independent samples t-test.

Maximum: The largest value in the dataset.

Mean: The 'average'. A measure of central tendency. The sum of the values divided by the number of values given.

Median: A measure of central tendency. The middle value of a set of values.

Minimum: The smallest value in the dataset.

Missing: A legitimate response was not given.

Multiple linear regression: An extension of simple linear regression to include more independent variables, which could be continuous or categorical (or a mixture of both).

Multistage random sampling: Take a random sample of large units where the population is grouped, then take a random sample of individuals from within those units.

Mutually exclusive categories: Categories within a research question which participants can only appear in one, and appearing in one, precludes them from appearing in any other category. For example, if the question was 'What age group do you belong?', and the possible responses were 18 to 24, 25 to 34, 35 to 44, 45 to 64, 65+, participants could only belong to one category because their actual age can only fit into one of the groups given.

Mutually exclusive events: Two events are mutually exclusive if, when one occurs, the other cannot happen.

Negative predictive value: The proportion of participants who are test negative and who are also disease negative.

Negatively skewed: Data where the majority of the observations are at the upper end of the range. If the median is greater than the mean, the data are skewed to the left.

Nominal scale: A categorical variable that is not ordered.

Normal distribution: It is the basis of many statistical tests and modelling. It is characteristically bell shaped with the mean and median at the centre of the distribution. Sixty-eight percent of data are contained within one standard deviation of the mean and approximately 95% are contained within two standard deviations of the mean.

Normal probability plot: It plots the standardised observed cumulative probability against the standardised expected cumulative probability of a linear regression. Assumptions of Normality are not violated when the plot shows a diagonal line.

NPV: See negative predictive value.

Null hypothesis (H_0):   Hypothesis of no difference or no relationship which is the underlying assumption when carrying out a significance test. It takes the general form: There is no difference or relationship in the population from which the samples are drawn. An alternative hypothesis must also be set up.

Numerator: The number of participants who have a given characteristic. For example, the number of females in a birth cohort.

Odds: The probability that an individual will have an event/disease/condition divided by the probability that they will not have the event/disease/condition.

Odds ratio: The ratio of the odds of an event/disease/condition amongst those with a given characteristic, to the odds of an event/disease/condition for those without the characteristic of interest.

One-way ANOVA: In its simplest form one-way analysis of variance is used as an analogue to the independent samples t-test to compare means when there are more than two groups. There are two assumptions underlying this test. The first is that the data come from a Normal distribution within group. The second is that the variances of the groups are equal.

OR: See odds ratio.

Ordinal scale: A variable where there is some order to the categories.

Outcome: See dependent variable.

Paired t-test: A parametric test used to compare means in matched or paired data. For example, where the data are before and after (comparing blood pressure before and after exercise) or where there are data from matched cases and controls. Assumption: the changes/differences are Normally distributed.

Parametric test: A statistical test that makes a distributional assumption.

Pearson's correlation coefficient: Used to discover how closely related two continuous variables are to one another by quantifying the strength and direction of the linear relationship.

Percent: The percentage of the total number in the dataset with a given response. Calculated by (numerator/denominator) $\times$ 100.

Percentile: It divides the distribution into one-hundredths.

Per protocol analysis: Analysis of only those in a randomised controlled trial who complied with the protocol.

Pie charts: A method for showing visually a variable that has a number of mutually exclusive categories. The larger the slice, the greater the percentage of the dataset falls into that category. A pie chart should not be used to display data from dichotomous variables.

Placebo: Inactive treatment sometimes used in randomised controlled trials which looks and tastes exactly like the active treatment.

Population: The set of all objects/people/events that we are interested in knowing about.

Positively skewed: Data where the majority of the observations are at the lower end of the range. If the median is less than the mean, the data are skewed to the right.

Positive predictive value: The proportion of participants who are test positive and who are also disease positive.

PPV: See positive predictive value.

Probability: The proportion of times an event would occur in the long run.

Proportion: The number with a given characteristic divided by the total number who have non-missing data.

Protocol: A document describing the aims and rationale of a study. In addition it usually describes how the resulting data are to be analysed. Some studies may require a clinical protocol, describing the procedures to be adhered to with regard to patients and the intervention/their treatment.

P-value: The result of a significance test. The probability of getting a difference as large or larger as that observed if there was no underlying difference or association in the population.

Questionnaire: A tool used for collecting data. It can be set up so that the respondent can self complete, alternately the researcher can read the questions to the respondent and complete the questionnaire. Questionnaires can be printed and completed on paper or programmed onto a computer. If questionnaires are computer aided, checks can be incorporated to reduce the number of inconsistent answers within respondent or values that are beyond the possible range. For example, a respondent reporting that they are 3m tall.

If possible, it is better to use a questionnaire that has been used in previous research. The questionnaire may have been used in a pilot study before it was used in the main research project, meaning the questions would have been tested and altered as necessary.

Quota sampling: A way of sample selection according to the characteristics of the people in the population, so the required number of people with the given combinations of characteristics are included in the study.

Randomised controlled trial: An experimental/interventional study design whereby participants are randomly assigned to a treatment group.

Random variation: Variation in data for unknown reasons. Random variation is often more evident in smaller datasets.

Ranking: Putting data in order of magnitude.

Receiver operating curve: A plot of sensitivity versus 1-specificity. It enables the point that maximises sensitivity and specificity to be identified. The optimum specificity and sensitivity is at the point that on the curve is closest to the top left of the curve.

Reference category: The category within a variable that the other categories are compared to in regression analyses.

Relative risk: The risk of an event in group 1 divided by the risk of the event in group 2.

Residuals: The difference between the observed values of the dependent variable and those resulting from the regression modelling.

Right skew: See positively skewed.

Risk: It is used in cohort or prospective studies. The proportion of persons in a given population, initially free of a disease who develop it within a specified time.

Risk difference: The difference between two proportions.

ROC: See receiver operating curve.

RR: See relative risk.

Sample: A group of individuals taken from a population to derive inferences about the population.

Sampling frame: The list from which a sample is drawn.

Scatterplot: Graphical representation of two continuous variables to show how they are related to one another.

SD: See standard deviation.

SE: See standard error.

Sensitivity: The number who are disease/event/condition positive and test positive divided by the number who are disease/event/condition positive. This equates to the proportion of positives that are test positive.

Significance test: A statistical test to investigate an hypothesis relating to differences or relationships between variables.

Sign test: A non-parametric analogue of the paired t-test.

Simple linear regression: It is used to investigate the nature of a relationship between two continuous variables, where one is regarded as predicting the other, rather than the strength.

Simple random sampling: All members of the population have an equal chance of being a member of the sample.

Slope: The increase in y (the dependent variable) when x (the independent variable) increases by one unit.

Spearman's rank correlation coefficient: The non-parametric analogue of Pearson's correlation. It gives a coefficient called rho (ρ), which is interpreted in the same way as Pearson's correlation coefficient.

Specificity: The number who are disease/event/condition negative and test negative divided by the number who are disease/event/condition negative. This equates to the proportion of negatives that are test negative.

SPSS: A computer program used for statistically analysing data.

Standard deviation: A measure of dispersion in the same units as the mean and the observations. It measures the average difference between the individual observations and the overall mean.

Standard error: An estimate of the precision of a sample estimate and is the standard deviation of the estimate.

Statistical significance: Having a p-value <0.05.

Stem and leaf plot: A way of displaying a continuous variable to show its distribution. They are not normally used in reports/papers, but are useful when exploring the data. The stem shows the leading digit(s) and the leaf shows the final digit.

Stratified random sampling: Divide the population into groups, for example by age or sex. Take a random sample from each group. Each group will have the same number in the sample.

Summary statistics: Statistics used to characterise the dataset in question. Usually they consist of measures of central tendency (and appropriate measure of dispersion) for continuous data or numbers with characteristics and associated percentages for categorical data.

Systematic allocation: For example, allocating treatments alternately (or another systematic way). The system is known, so is open to abuse, for example, not recruiting some potential participants because that treatment is not wanted for that participant.

Systematic sampling: Selecting a study sample using an identifiable method which means that potential participants do not have an equal probability of being in the sample.

Test statistic: A statistic that is calculated as part of a statistical test. The more extreme the test statistic (positive or negative if a two-sided test has been set up), the smaller the p-value.

Two-way ANOVA: An analysis of variance in which two factors are incorporated at the same time. The same result would be obtained by doing a multiple linear regression with two independent variables.

Valid: Responses where a legitimate answer is given.

Valid Percent: The percentage of the valid data with a given response.

Variable: Attributes that characterise members of a population and which may vary from individual to individual. For example, height, weight, sex.

Variance: A measure of dispersion of a variable. The mean square of the difference between values of a given variable and the mean for that variable. For a sample, instead of dividing by the number of observations as with the mean, divide by the number of observations minus one, that is n−1. The variance is not in the same units as the variable in question so it is of limited practical use.

Wilcoxon matched pairs test: A non-parametric test analogous to the paired t-test.

X-axis: The horizontal axis on a graph.

Y-axis: The vertical axis on a graph.

REFERENCES

Altman, D.G. (1991) *Practical Statistics for Medical Research*. London: Chapman and Hall.

Altman, D.G. and Bland, J.M. (1994) 'Diagnostic tests 1: sensitivity and specificity', *BMJ*, 308: 1552.

Altman, D.G. and Matthews, J.N.S. (1996) 'Interaction 1: Heterogeneity of effects', *BMJ*, 313: 486.

Australian Bureau of Statistics (2007) www.abs.gov.au/websitedbs/d3310114.nsf/Home/census   Accessed November 2007.

Aveyard, P., Brown, K., Saunders, C., Alexander, A., Johnstone, E., Munafò, M.R. and Murphy, M. (2007) 'Weekly versus basic smoking cessation support in primary care: a randomised controlled trial', *Thorax*, 62: 898–903.

Bayley, N. (1993) *Manual for the Bayley Scales of Infant Development II*. San Antonio TX: Psychological Corporation.

Benaim, C., Pérennou, D.A., Villy, J., Rousseaux, M. and Pelissier, J.Y. (1999) 'Validation of a standardized assessment of postural control in stroke patients', *Stroke*, 30: 1862–8.

Bergström, G., Bodin, L. Bertilsson, H. and Jensen, I.B. (2007) 'Risk factors for new episodes of sick leave due to neck or back pain in a working population. A prospective study with an eighteen-month and a three-year follow-up', *Occupational and Environmental Medicine*, 64: 279–87.

Bland, M. (2000) *An Introduction to Medical Statistics* (3rd edition). Oxford: Oxford University Press.

Cooper, R., Blell, M., Hardy, R., Black, S., Pollard, T.M., Wadsworth, M.E.J., Pearce, M.S. and Kuh, D. (2006) 'Validity of age at menarche self-reported in adulthood', *Journal of Epidemiology and Community Health*, 60: 993–7.

Covic, T., Roufeil, L. and Dziurawiec, S. (2007) 'Community beliefs about childhood obesity: its causes, consequences and potential solutions', *Journal of Public Health*, 29 (2): 123–31.

De Tychey, C., Briançon, S., Lighezzolo, J., Spitz, E., Kabuth, B., de luigi, V., Messembourg, C., Girvan, F., Rosati, A., Thockler, A. and Vincent, S. (2008) 'Quality of life, postnatal depression and baby gender', *Journal of Clinical Nursing*, 17: 312–22.

Donner, A. and Klar, N. (2000) *Design and Analysis of Cluster Randomization Trials in Health Research*. London: Arnold.

Evans, J., Heron, J., Francomb, H., Oke, S. and Golding, J. (2001) 'Cohort study of depressed mood during pregnancy and after childbirth', *BMJ*, 323 (7307): 257–60.

Freeman, J.V., Walters, S.J. and Campbell, M.J. (2008) *How to Display Data*. Oxford. BMJ Books, Blackwell.

Graff, M.J.L., Vernooij-Dassen, M.J.M., Thijssen, M., Dekker, J., Hoefnagels, W.H.L. and Olde Rikkert, M.G.M. (2006) 'Community based occupational therapy for patients with dementia and their care givers: randomised controlled trial', *BMJ*, 333 (7580): 1196–201.

International Association of Athletics Federations (2008) Statistics – Men – One Mile. www.iaaf.org/statistics/records/gender=M/allrecords/discipline=MILE/index.html Accessed January 2008.

Johansson, S.E., Konlaan, B.B. and Bygren, L.O. (2001) 'Sustaining habits of attending cultural events and maintenance of health: a longitudinal study', *Health Promotion International*, 16: 229–34.

Johnson, A.H., Peacock, J.L., Greenough, A., Marlow, N., Limb, E.S., Marston, L. and Calvert, S.A. for the United Kingdom Oscillation Study Group (2002) 'High-frequency oscillatory ventilation for the prevention of chronic lung disease of prematurity', *New England Journal of Medicine*, 347 (9): 633–42.

Johnson, S., Marlow, N., Wolke, D., Davidson, L., Marston, L., O'Hare, A., Peacock, J. and Schulte, J. (2004) 'Validation of a Parent report measure of cognitive development in very preterm infants', *Developmental Medicine and Child Neurology*, 46 (6): 389–97.

Kirkwood, B.R. and Sterne, J.A.C. (2003) *Essential Medical Statistics*. Oxford: Blackwell Publishing.

Lacey, R.J., Lewis, M. and Sim, J. (2007) 'Piecework, musculoskeletal pain and the impact of workplace psychosocial factors', *Occupational Medicine*, 57 (6): 430–7.

Maguire, H., Dale, J.W., McHugh, T.D., Butcher, P.D., Gillespie, S.H., Costetsos, A., Al-Ghusein, H., Holland, R., Dickens, A., Marston, L., Wilson, P., Pitman, R., Strachan, D., Drobniewski, F.A. and Banerjee, D.K. (2002) 'Molecular epidemiology of tuberculosis in London 1995–7 showing low rate of active transmission', *Thorax*, 57: 617–22.

Mahoney, F.I. and Barthel, D.W. (1965) 'Functional evaluation: The Barthel Index', *Maryland State Medical Journal*, 14: 61–5.

Marston, L., Peacock, J.L., Calvert, S.A., Greenough, A. and Marlow, N. (2007) 'Factors affecting vocabulary acquisition at age two in children born 23–28 weeks gestation', *Developmental Medicine and Child Neurology*, 49 (8): 591–6.

Marston, L., Peacock, J.L., Yu, K., Brocklehurst, P., Calvert, S.A., Greenough, A. and Marlow, N. (2009) 'Comparing methods of analysing datasets with small clusters: case studies using four paediatric datasets', *Paediatric and Perinatal Epidemiology*, 23 (4): 380–92.

Melchior, M., Roquelaure, Y., Evanoff, B., Chastang, J.F., Ha, C., Imbernon, E., Goldberg, M., Leclerc, A. and the Pays de la Loire Study Group (2006) 'Why are manual workers at high risk of upper limb disorders? The role of physical work factors in a random sample of workers in France (the Pays de la Loire study)', *Occupational and Environmental Medicine*, 63: 754–61.

Moore, H., Summerbell, C.D., Greenwood, D.C., Tovey, P., Griffiths, J., Henderson, M., Hesketh, K., Woolgar, S. and Adamson, A.J. (2003) 'Improving management of obesity in primary care: cluster randomised trial', *BMJ*, 327: 1085–8.

Mussaffi, H., Omer, R., Prais, D., Mei-Zahav, M., Weiss-Kasirer, T., Botzer, Z. and Blau, H. (2007) 'Computerised paediatric asthma quality of life questionnaires in routine care', *Archives of Disease in Childhood*, 92: 678–82.

Ng, G.Y.T., Derry, C., Marston, L., Choudhury, M., Holmes, K. and Calvert, S.A. (2008) 'Reduction in ventilator-induced lung injury improves outcome in congenital diaphragmatic hernia?', *Pediatric Surgery International*, 24: 145–50.

Office for National Statistics (2001) The UK Population by Ethnic Group. www.statistics. gov.uk/statbase/Expodata/Spreadsheets/D6588.xls   Accessed November 2007.

Office for National Statistics (2007a) Census Home. www.statistics.gov.uk/census/default. asp   Accessed November 2007.

Office for National Statistics (2007b) Birth Statistics. www.statistics.gov.uk/downloads/theme_population/FM1_35/FM1_No35.pdf   Accessed January 2008.

Office for National Statistics (2007c) Mortality Statistics. www.statistics.gov.uk/downloads/theme_health/Dh1_38_2005/DH1_No_38.pdf   Accessed January 2008.

Office for National Statistics (2007d) Health Statistics Quarterly 36. www.statistics.gov.uk/downloads/theme_health/HSQ36.pdf   Accessed January 2008.

Öhlander, E., Vikström, M., Lindström, M. and Sundquist, K. (2006) 'Neighbourhood non-employment and daily smoking: a population-based study of women and men in Sweden', *European Journal of Public Health*, 16: 78–84.

Palaniappan, U., Jacobs Starkey, L., O'Loughlin, J. and Gray-Donald, K. (2001) 'Fruit and vegetable consumption is lower and saturated fat intake is higher among Canadians reporting smoking', *The Journal of Nutrition*, 131: 1952–8.

Parry, G., Van Cleemput, P., Peters, J., Walters, S., Thomas, K. and Cooper, C. (2007) 'Health status of Gypsies and Travellers in England', *Journal of Epidemiology and Community Health*, 61:198–204.

Paterson, C. (1996) 'Measuring outcomes in primary care: a patient generated measure, MYMOP, compared with the SF-36 health survey', *BMJ*, 312 (7037): 1016–20.

Peacock, J.L. and Kerry, S.M. (2007) *Presenting Medical Statistics from Proposal to Publication: A Step-by-Step Guide*. Oxford: Oxford University Press.

Ramrakha, S., Caspi, A., Dickson, N., Moffitt, T.E. and Paul, C. (2000) 'Psychiatric disorders and risky sexual behaviour in young adulthood: cross sectional study in birth cohort', *BMJ*, 321: 263–6.

Rudd, A.G., Wolfe, C.D.A., Tilling, K. and Beech, R. (1997) 'Randomised controlled trial to evaluate early discharge scheme for patients with stroke', *BMJ*, 315: 1039–44.

Samanic, C.M., Kogevinas, M., Silverman, D.T. Serra, C., Malats, N., Real, F.X., Carrato, A., García-Closas, R., Sala, M., Leoreta, J., Rothman, N. and Dosemeci, M. (2008) 'Occupation and bladder cancer in a hospital-based case–control study in Spain', *Occupational and Environmental Medicine*, 65: 347–53.

Saxena, S., Ambler, G., Cole, T.J. and Majeed, A. (2004) 'Ethnic group differences in overweight and obese children and young people in England: cross sectional survey', *Archives of Disease in Childhood*, 89: 30–6.

Sofi, F., Capalbo, A., Pucci, N., Giuliattini, J., Condino, F., Alessandri, F., Abbate, R., Gensini, G.F. and Califano, S. (2008) 'Cardiovascular evaluation, including resting and exercise electrocardiography, before participation in competitive sports: cross sectional study', *BMJ*, 337 (7661): 88–92.

SPSS Inc (2007) SPSS Technical Support for Students. http://support.spss.com/Student/Studentdefault.asp   Accessed September 2007.

Stein, M.S., Maskill, D. and Marston, L. (2009) 'Impact of visual-spatial neglect on stroke functional outcomes, discharge destination and maintenance of improvement post-discharge', *British Journal of Occupational Therapy*, 72: 219–25.

Stroke Association (2008) The Stroke Association – Neglect. www.stroke.org.uk/information/all_about_stroke/rehabilitation/performing_daily_activities/neglect.html Accessed April 2008.

Tappin, D., Brooke, H., Ecob, R. and Gibson, A. (2002) 'Used infant mattresses and sudden infant death syndrome in Scotland: case-control study', *BMJ*, 325: 1007.

Thorpe, L.E., Gwynn, R.C., Mandel-Ricci, J., Roberts, S., Tsoi, B., Berman, L., Porter, K., Ostchega, Y., Curtain, L.R., Montaquila, J., Mohadjer, L. and Frieden, T.R. (2006) 'Study design and participation rates of the New York City Health and Nutrition Examination Survey, 2004', *Preventing Chronic Disease*, 3 (3): A94.

Tinetti, M.E. (1986) 'Performance-oriented assessment of mobility problems in elderly patients', *Journal of the American Geriatric Society*, 34: 119–26.

US Census Bureau (2007) www.census.gov   Accessed November 2007.

Vinkers, D.J., Gussekloo, J., Stek, M.L., Westendorp, R.G.J. and van der Mast, R.C. (2004) 'Temporal relation between depression and cognitive impairment in old age: prospective population based study', *BMJ*, 329: 881–3.

Wilson, L.M., Roden, P.W., Taylor, Y. and Marston, L. (2008) 'The effectiveness of Origami on overall hand function after injury: a pilot controlled trial', *British Journal of Hand Therapy*, 13: 12–20.

Wood, S.A. and Lutman, M.E. (2004) 'Relative benefits of linear analogue and advanced digital hearing aids', *International Journal of Audiology*, 43 (3):144–55.

Zhu, T., Buoling, F., Shiushing, W., Won, C. and Shu-Hong, Z. (2004) 'A comparison of smoking behaviors among medical and other college students in China', *Health Promotion International*, 19 (2): 189–96.

INDEX

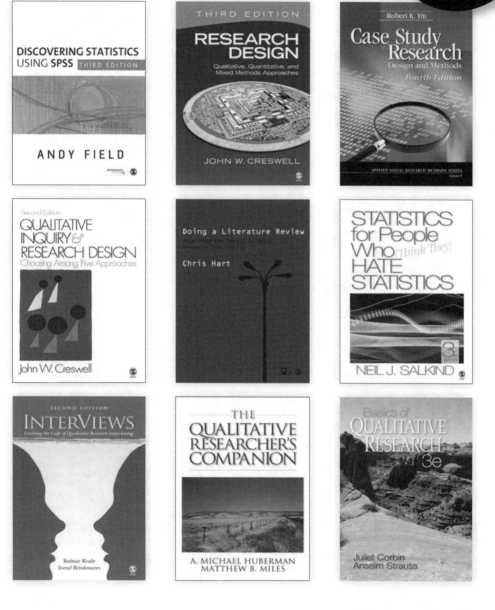
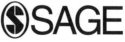

The Qualitative Research Kit

Edited by Uwe Flick

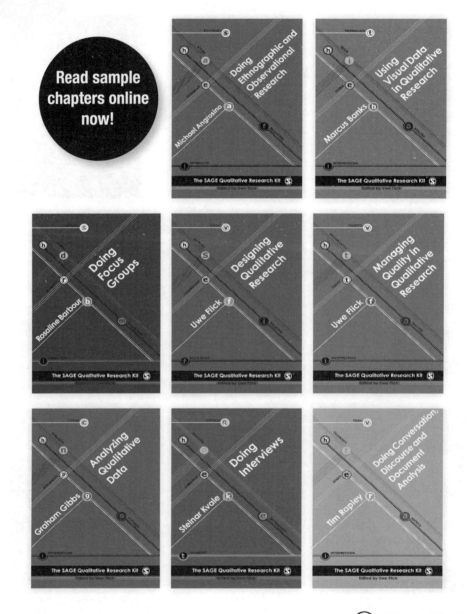

Read sample chapters online now!

Doing Ethnographic and Observational Research — Michael Angrosino — The SAGE Qualitative Research Kit — Edited by Uwe Flick

Using Visual Data in Qualitative Research — Marcus Banks — The SAGE Qualitative Research Kit — Edited by Uwe Flick

Doing Focus Groups — Rosaline Barbour — The SAGE Qualitative Research Kit — Edited by Uwe Flick

Designing Qualitative Research — Uwe Flick — The SAGE Qualitative Research Kit — Edited by Uwe Flick

Managing Quality in Qualitative Research — Uwe Flick — The SAGE Qualitative Research Kit — Edited by Uwe Flick

Analyzing Qualitative Data — Graham Gibbs — The SAGE Qualitative Research Kit — Edited by Uwe Flick

Doing Interviews — Steinar Kvale — The SAGE Qualitative Research Kit — Edited by Uwe Flick

Doing Conversation, Discourse and Document Analysis — Tim Rapley — The SAGE Qualitative Research Kit — Edited by Uwe Flick

www.sagepub.co.uk

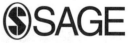

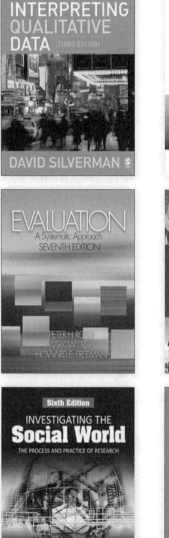
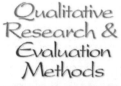
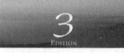
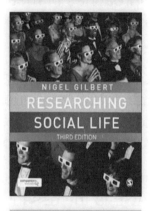
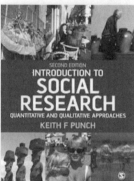
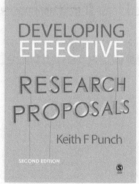
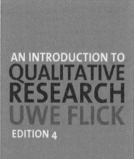
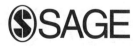

Supporting researchers for more than forty years

Research methods have always been at the core of SAGE's publishing. Sara Miller McCune founded SAGE in 1965 and soon after she published SAGE's first methods book, *Public Policy Evaluation*. A few years later, she launched the Quantitative Applications in the Social Sciences series – affectionately known as the 'little green books'.

Always at the forefront of developing and supporting new approaches in methods, SAGE published early groundbreaking texts and journals in the fields of qualitative methods and evaluation.

Today, more than forty years and two million little green books later, SAGE continues to push the boundaries with a growing list of more than 1,200 research methods books, journals, and reference works across the social, behavioural, and health sciences.

From qualitative, quantitative and mixed methods to evaluation, SAGE is the essential resource for academics and practitioners looking for the latest in methods by leading scholars.

www.sagepublications.com

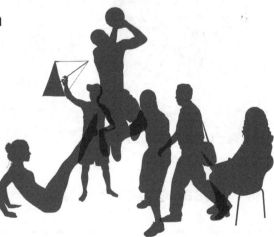

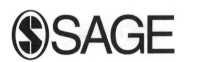